Nutrition food

Healthy and Longer life Secrets

Copyright

Copyright © 2022 by Meher Afshan

Introduction

Name of the author: Meher Afshan (M.sc)

My name is Meher Afshan. I have a master's degree in Genetics from Karachi University of Pakistan. I have done a certificate course in I.T and Financial Accounting. I was a trained teacher and Principal. I quit my job in 2017 and have been working in the online field ever since. I started blogging two years ago and I have four YouTube channels. I have self-published four books e-books and three low content books on Amazon Kindle. My upcoming books are four e-books, low content books and, children's books. Before that, I wrote an article about my student life in various magazines and newspapers.

I have worked as a compere and a host on Radio Pakistan Karachi in an evening transmission Sar-e Sham.
I am from Pakistan but my books and other materials are for all countries.
I work as a blogger by the end of March 2019.
My new blog URL is https://learnandearnafs.blogspot.com.

I have four YouTube channels but now working on two channels, links are in my blog. I will start the kid's YouTube channel soon and after that, I will create an app. I love writing and love to work as a YouTube creator and planning to create audio courses.
My hobbies are reading, writing, listening music, create designing, and watching good videos. Now lack of time I cannot manage reading time and watching time.
I hope you will like this book and other books and all you will corporate with me. Write review, comment, like, and share if you can, happy to read any suggestions at the end of this book and on my blog post.

Contents

Chapter 1

Nutrition

Word nutrition means anything to eat or anything nourishing in solid or in liquid form that human or animals eat or drink to maintain life and growth to perform daily activity correctly, but all foodstuff are not good that human choose from to make up their diet, animal satisfies its daily requirement of food through natural selection. All foods that humans choose are not consists of essential nutrients such as carbohydrates, fat, protein, vitamins, mineral, and water. Carbohydrate foods also provide fiber, which acts as roughage and helps the gut wall to keep the food moving through it. You should include adequate starchy foods as a source of glucose.

Limit consumption of salt, too much sugar, alcohol, saturated fats.

Keep good immunity, vitamin C can help to control the immune system well. Avoid too much sugar. Researchers believe that sugar disturbs healthy bacteria. A nutritious meal keeps the body healthy inside and outside.

Carbohydrates, fats, proteins, mineral, and vitamins, which sustain life, generate energy and provide growth, maintenance, and health. All living organisms require food to carry on their life process, if we do not eat a day or two we become weak, food provides energy. Food is what we take in for strength and nutrition, it means not only the variety of food used but also the proportion in which it is needed and its utilization for a healthy body. Not whatever anyone eats necessary for eating healthy food, different foods have different effects on the body, so the knowledge of a balanced diet in all constituents of food in adequate proportion is important. Foods we eat provide energy and energy produce by carbohydrates and fats, bodybuilding by proteins, and body protection by Vitamins and minerals.

The foods, which we take, consist of the seven nutrition groups:

Carbohydrates, Fats, Proteins, Vitamins, Minerals, Water and Enzymes

Carbohydrates:

To perform a vital function of the body we need sufficient energy and chemical constituents for use in many different ways in the body. Carbohydrates supply 70 to 80% of the total energy requirement. Each gram of it provides 4 calories. Carbohydrates are the first and quick source of energy in our body. These are the fuel of our body because of the most direct source of energy. When we chew starchy bread, it tastes sweet. It has turned into sugar. The glucose formed by the digestion of the sugar and starches is absorbed into the blood through the walls of the intestine and finally carried to the liver. Sweet foods have turned into sugar our body uses simple sugar as its source of energy. 350 grams is stored in the form of glycogen in muscle and liver.

Carbohydrates contain elements such as carbon, hydrogen, and oxygen. The glucose absorbed helps to maintain the glucose level in the blood any excess convert to fat and is being stored. Carbohydrates are organic compounds found in potatoes, noodles, pasta, rice, bread slice, sweet potato, oats, yam, green bananas, and barley. Fruits provide simple sugar called fructose when molecules of sugars (glucose and fructose) to form a complex 2 sugar molecules called sucrose. Our daily use of sugar is sucrose from sugar cane. Lactose found in milk is also a 2-sugar molecule. Complex carbohydrates such as starch, cellulose, and glycogen are found from simple sugar molecules joins in a long chain, for example, starch, first broken down into glucose by digestion in our body, second glucose is oxidized in cells to yield energy during cellular respiration. Some carbohydrates like refined flour are increased insulin levels while legumes are slower.

Fats

Fats are the second source of energy. Fats contain carbon, hydrogen, and oxygen and are composed of fatty acids. In our daily meal, excess food in our body is stored in the form of fat. In our body during starvation the absence of sugars, fats are broken down to release energy. One mole of fat produces 9000 calories of energy. Each gm of it gives 9 calories. It is utilize as the carrier of fat-soluble Vitamin A, D, E, and K protection for the heart and brain, padding around the organs holding them in place, and absorbing the stocks.

Fatty substance in food contains oils and fats, oils remain in liquid on room temperature while fats remain in solid on room temperature. Most of the fats made up of smaller chemical units such as fatty acids and glycerol. Vegetable oils such as soya bean, corn, mustard oils, and sunflower seeds oils remain liquid at room temperature while cottonseeds oil remains solid at room temperature. We can divide fatty acids into four types; saturated, mono-saturated, poly saturated, and Trans- fats.

Monounsaturated fatty acids are known as good fats, it decreases the risk of heart disease and also helps of reduce type 2 diabetes and overall health, lower LDL cholesterol level and increase HDL, prevent abnormal heart rhythms, lower blood pressure lower triglycerides and fight inflammation, prevent atherosclerosis, example are Olives, peanut butter, avocado, nuts, canola, sesame oil

Polyunsaturated fat is good for overall health as monounsaturated fat. It found in pumpkin seeds, sesame, sunflower, flaxseed, fatty fish such as salmon, trout, tuna, and herring fish oil and mackerel fish, tofu, soymilk walnut. **Omega-3 fatty acids**, a diet rich in omega-3 may help to support a healthy pregnancy, battle fatigue, balance mood, sharpen memory, reduce risk heart diseases, ease arthritis, inflammatory skin condition, joint pain, protect against memory loss, prevent and reduce of symptoms of depression.

Saturated fatty acids: A fat contains a high proportion of fatty acid. A fat that contains only saturated fatty acids is remaining in solid at room temperature, **scientist said that saturated fats can raise your bad cholesterol and put you at higher risk of heart diseases. It can raise LDL.**

Saturated fats found in red meat(beef, pork, and lamb), butter, palm oil, coconut oil, red meat fat, solid shortening, lard, cheese, cream, and cocoa butter.

Full fat milk raises the level of cholesterol in the blood. However, the latest research shows that if cutting down all saturated fats then these foods are good. It's important to add right foods such as vegetable oil like olive oil in place of butter to help lower cholesterol and reduce risk of diseases but do not replace refined carbohydrates for example junk foods or in breakfast item replacing pastry because refined carbohydrate or sugary foods on have a similar negative effect on the body as saturated fat.

Unsaturated fatty acids: These acids remain in liquid at room temperature like groundnuts; safflower oil and sesame oil do not increase blood cholesterol level. Refined oils are good for health, it improves the quality and taste, these oils are free from odor and color it removes free fatty acid and rancid material from it.

Unsaturated fats are considered healthy fats and are good for health, these fats help reduce high blood cholesterol levels and the risk of heart diseases, Help to manage mood, fight fatigue and help to control weight, for example, fatty fish, peanuts, nuts, and seeds, olives, avocados and its oil, vegetable oil such as corn, canola, sunflower, and refined olive oil.

Dietary fats and cholesterol: Cholesterol level is dependent upon dietary fats, cholesterol is not bad but too much is not good for everyone's health, there are two types of cholesterol, good and bad. HDL cholesterol is a good type of cholesterol found in our blood while LDL is a bad type of cholesterol, for best health LDL, should be low and HDL should be a high level of cholesterol to protect against heart diseases or strokes. As export, say limiting intake of saturated fat can help to improve health, 10% of daily calories.

Sources of dietary fats
There are two ways to get dietary fats: **Animals and vegetables**

Animal fats: animal fats are poor sources of fatty acids and remain in solid form at room temperature but they are a good source of Vitamin A and D such as red meat fat, butter, and fish oil, Oysters, Tuna, sardines, anchovies, mussels, halibut, mussels, and mackerel.

Vegetable fats: Vegetable fats are in the form of liquid, examples are corn, canola, sunflower, refined olive oil. Parents usually recognize these foods for kids like candy, donuts, sugary breakfast cereals, fruit drinks, cookies, ice cream, chicken nuggets, lunchmeat, hot dog, French fries, potato chips, and other junk foods full of sugar and highly processed foods. Small amounts of naturally avoid to do so as experts say.

Proteins

Proteins are large organic molecules that contain hydrogen, oxygen, carbon, nitrogen, and sulfur and one mole of the protein produce about 4000 calories of energy however, their main role is in building material in the body. Amino acids play a building block role in protein, there are twenty kinds of amino acids, and these combine in different ways to make different kinds and a great variety of proteins. The number of amino acids combined in most protein molecules ranges, 300 to 3000. Proteins are necessary for life, the cell nucleus and protoplasm of everybody are made of proteins, our daily activity needs energy, our energy requirements change due to our activities performed by the body and it also depends on a person's weight, sex, and age.

The function of proteins in our body to provide energy in the presence of sugar and fats and stimulate metabolism, material for growth, proteins make enzymes and ferments concerned in digestion, transformed into carbohydrates, which under certain condition may synthesized to fat.

Red blood cells contain important proteins, hemoglobin for the transport of oxygen in our body. The protein we eat in our food, for example, meat and egg albumin are broken in our body into amino acids, and from these, our cells make their type of proteins. A high-quality protein intake has increased metabolic rate, reduce appetite, help build muscle, and preserve muscle during weight loss. One-sixth of the bodyweight contains proteins, one-third in the muscles, one fifth in cartilage and bone one-tenth in the skin, and remaining in tissues and body fluid.

Sources of protein;

Two major sources of proteins are **animal and plant**.

Animal sources /100 gm mutton 18.5 fish 21.5 and milk, yogurt, Chicken breast, eggs, milk are higher Eggs, chicken breast, cottage cheese, and liver.

Plant sources are beans, lentils, pulses, almonds, broccoli, oats, yellow sweet corn, potato, lentils, green Pease, carrot, dark green vegetables, lose-leafed vegetables like broccoli, cauliflower and Nuts are black beans, almond they help in growth and repair of body parts, means healing; they also make structures like hair, muscles, and nails. New cells, red blood cells being form all the time in the body. Inadequacy proteins lead low growth and weaken our immune system.

Vitamin

Vitamin is a complex organic compound required for normal growth and nutrition but an organism needs it in small quantities for the proper function of its metabolism. Vitamin does not play any role as a source of energy but they are essential for life, absence of vitamins in our body results in serious malfunction. We can say vitamin is of two types; fat-soluble or water-soluble, and fat-soluble are vitamin A, D, E, and K, and water-soluble are vitamin C, and vitamin B Complex. Most of the vitamins cannot synthesize by the body but are found naturally in the foods that can be obtained by animals and plants.

Vitamin A;

It is fat-soluble, it can be stored in the body and 90% of it is stored in the liver. This Vitamin is real life, a life-giving vitamin, this vitamin is essential for normal vision, immune function, and Mc Collum and Davis at John Hopkins University in America discovered reproduction skin Vitamin when they were isolating growth factor in yolk and butter. The first time in 1930, it chemically synthesized. It protects from lung cancer, vision, drying skin issues, essential for skeletal growth, anti-protected by protecting the body from microbes, role-play in the immunological defense mechanism of the body.

Absence of Vitamin A: An adequate amount in our body causes night blindness eye diseases such as glaucoma and cataract and drying of the skin. Retinol find only in animal origin.

Sources of vitamin A: The main source is Cod liver oil, which also helps heart and kidney function properly antioxidant, naturally found in Apple, Mangoes, milk, Carrots, tuna fish, fish liver oil, sweet potatoes, carrot, spinach, cauliflower, eggs, Loquat, Pumpkin, Peaches, Pomegranates, Yellow and Red bell pepper, Tomatoes, Plums, Winter squashes, Broccoli, Kale, Lettuce, and Cod liver oil. The cod liver has used for centuries even though Vitamin A was not discovered, in Romans and Greeks; night blindness was alleviated by eating liver. Liver, egg yolk, milk, butter and fish, dark green vegetables such as cabbage, broccoli, mint, coriander, spinach, mango ripe, yellow-colored carrots, papaya, pumpkin

Consumption of excess of Vitamin A causes headache, irritation, fatigue, vomiting, nausea, and anorexia.

Vitamin B;

This vitamin is a complex of many vitamins called Vitamin B Complex such as B1 sources of thiamine include in, B2, B3, B4, B5, B6, B12, and others. The fact is, in our large intestine certain bacteria can be prepared due to some type of B-complex vitamins. Foods contain vitamin B; are whole grain such as barley, millet and brown rice, broccoli, kale, spinach, almond, sunflower seeds, beans, lentils, eggs, milk, cheese, poultry, fish, chicken, bananas, yellow and red bell pepper red meat, citrus fruits, bananas, avocado, red challis, pomegranates.

Vitamin B1 helps to maintain heart and nerve function. Deficiency of this causes anorexia, muscle weakness, and nerve damages, these Vitamins are present in green beans, sweet potatoes, milk, eggs, wheat grains, mushrooms, almond, red meat.

Vitamin B2 also called Riboflavin. Its role is promoting blood cells and body metabolism.

Food sources of Vitamin B2

 Asparagus, peaches, brown bread, liver, boiled eggs, milk, dark leafy vegetables, meat, chicken, bread, almonds, fortified cereals, and cooked beef are the main sources of this Vitamin.

 Insufficient Vitamin B2 causes cracked lips, sore tongue, and affects normal growth.

Vitamin B3

Niacin found in Vitamin B3, which helps in maintaining the cardiovascular and metabolism system in the body helps to balance cholesterol levels.

Vitamin B3

 Liver and chicken breast are the main source of niacin, salmon and tuna fish, pork and turkey, ground beef, pineapple, mushrooms, pear, plum, strawberries, chicken, eggs, and dairy products.

Deficiency of vitamin B3

occurs vomiting and diarrhea, fatigue, depression, swollen mouth, bright red tongue, headache, disorientation, inflammation of the skin due to sunlight, and apathy.

Vitamin B4

Vitamin B4 is also defined as adenine and water-soluble, it is absorbed from the upper part of the small intestine, though the body does not store this vitamin.

Vitamin B5

Vitamin B5 also called pantothenic acid and it supports the adrenal glands, which reduces stress and anxiety levels. It is important for our life and necessary to make blood cells also help to convert food into energy.

Vitamin B5 is found in meat, chicken, pork, liver and kidney, salmon, shellfish, lobster, beef, turkey duck, whole grain bread.

Deficiency of Vitamin B5

It is rare but may include symptoms like vomiting, insomnia, depression, fatigue, stomach pains, feet burning, and upper respiratory infections.

Vitamin B6

It also called pyridoxine and water-soluble vitamin, essential for several body functions.

Food source of vitamin B6

Whole grain cereals, fish, pork, eggs, brown bread, sweet potatoes, chicken, turkey, green beans, and soya beans are the example of this. Vitamin B6 is important to carbohydrate metabolism and the creation of red blood cells. Keep to control in disorders of the nervous system.

Vitamin B9

This vitamin is also known as Folate an essential nutrient that plays a role in cell growth and also takes part in the formation of DNA.

Vitamin B12

It is also called folate our body needs folate to make DNA and other genetic material. It is also required for body cells to divide.

Vitamin B12

The main food sources are liver, chicken, beef; fish, salmon, tuna fish, fortified breakfast cereal, low-fat milk, and eggs are examples of Vitamin B12. The body absorbs only as much as it needs and excess passes through urine. Vitamin B12 is important for red blood cells; helps to prevent a type of anemia called megaloblastic anemia in which the growth of red blood cells increases than normal and does not function properly.

Symptoms of deficiency of Vitamin B12

It includes mouth ulcers, pin, and needles paraesthesia, memory loss, disturbed vision, constipation, loss of appetite, gas, diarrhea, sore and red tongue, extreme tiredness, lack of energy, shortness of breath, pale skin and muscles weakness, neurological problems which effect of the nervous system

Vitamin C

 is water-soluble and the body cannot store this for long. The chemical name is Ascorbic Acid, required for the building of connective tissue inside the human body, vital overall health and to beautify skin due to antioxidants, it helps to create collagen, is a type of connective tissues that keeps our skin firm, protecting the skin from damages, and allows wounds to heal quickly. Smoking destroys Vitamin C, any kind of stress where an argument or fatigue, illness, or extremes of temperature depletes Vitamin C.

Vitamin C sources; Vitamin is found in Lemon, Tomatoes, Cherry, Water Melon, Berries; all Citrus Fruits contain Vitamin C, and this Vitamin also present in fresh vegetables such as Broccoli, Kali. Fruits and veggies should be fresh. Wash all utensils before using them for any purpose. Vitamin C is rich in helpful nutrients, In other words, it helps in building immunity. That food rich in vitamin C help an individual to develop resistance against infection and helps to eliminate harmful free radicals that cause certain cancer. vitamin C deficiency contains; Gum bleeding, (disease scurvy), Scurvy causes fatigue, corkscrew hair, poor wound healing, several mental illnesses, smoking, and dialysis small red or purple spots on the skin, joint pain.

The advantage of Vitamin C: the physical body system needs good immunity to function well, or we will say immunity is that the main feature of a healthy body an honest system helps to stay one faraway from infection and diseases.

Vitamin D we will get vitamin D direct from the sun, Vitamin D, is required for the event of strong bones; it helps within the absorption of calcium, which makes the bone hard. Sun is that the main source of vitamin D. This vitamin also referred to as sunshine Vitamin, Sun may be a great source of vitamin D but those couldn't get vitamin D through the sun can eat many fish, mushrooms, eggs, wheat grain, liver, boiled eggs, milk, sunflower-seed oil, and seeds. Vitamin D is fighting against infection, acne, plant disease on the skin, for strong bones.

Deficiency of vitamin D Medical sources says that the signs and symptoms of vitamin D deficiency affecting on person's well being, depression Schizophrenia, asthma wheezing, type 1 diabetes thanks to the pancreas, high vital sign coronary heart condition, aches weakness Causes in children legs to become bowed, broken bones like osteoporosis and fractures. In other words, symptoms of vitamin D can explain during this way deficiency feeling tired, sleep changes, low mood, fatigue, pale skin and dark circle, back pain, streptococcal sore throat, loss of appetite, frequent cough and cold, muscle strength, week and aching bones. Vitamin E Vitamin E antioxidant makes skin beautiful protects from radical damage, perfect for acne removal, oil soluble.

Source of vitamin E;

Such as nuts, pomegranate, cherry, carrot, boiled eggs, red berries, oil-like sunflower-seed oil, and lots of other foods those have oil.

Vitamin K

Vitamin K is important to assist in clotting blood, healthy bones healing wounds and bruises, it's also produced by intestinal bacteria, deficiency of it dark circle and skin to seem dark and spider veins problem appears, include liver, milk, kale and cabbage, green leaves.

Symptoms of vitamin K deficiency;

Excessive bleeding when an individual is cut or wounded, hemorrhage disease of the newborn. Choline may be a vitamin found in some foods like milk, eggs, cucumber, walnut, cabbage, bananas, kale, turnip, green leaf lettuce, mustard green, parsley, cauliflower, fish, liver, meat, and peanuts but the body can develop this vitamin itself, it's important for the traditional brain, synthesis of neurotransmitters function and play a crucial role in somatic cell membranes.

Minerals

We also required certain inorganic substances in our food like Calcium, potassium, sodium, phosphorus, iron, iodine fluoride. Calcium is required for bones and teeth, vital for growing children. Foods source of calcium is milk, eggs, fruits, cheese, almonds, and green vegetables. Iron is extremely essential for the formation of hemoglobin (red cells within the blood), found in apple, spinach, mango, and many other foods. Iron deficiency may cause fatigue, low energy, and irritability. Potassium, chlorine (chloride), and sodium are important for nerve and muscle cells, found in body fluids. Phosphorus rich in fish, milk, oyster, cheese, and eggs, it found within the bones in sort of phosphate. It a constituent of body cells and serves to manage the metabolism of the body. Iodine is vital for thyroid hormone; absence of this makes deficiency of the hormone, rich in seafood. Fluoride helps to fight against the cavity.

Water

Water is important for the transport of nutrients and dehydration can cause a scarcity of energy. Water is extremely essential for our body, to process of digestion many substances circulated within the body as a watery solution within the blood. Our body uses water for all its cells, organs, and tissues to assist regulate its temperature and maintain other bodily functions. On day to day, our body loses much water, lost from our body through breathing, sweating, and urinating. It's vital to drink more water to balance lost water and rehydrate by drinking fluid and eating foods that contain water. Consistent with a cardiac specialist beverage at a particular time of the day can prevent an attack in the dark and therefore the early hour of the day.

Enzymes;

The process during which, insoluble starches of carbohydrates convert into soluble sugar within the presence of enzymes. Enzymes are liable for the chemical digestion of food in our body. When we eat, cut it into small pieces chew by the teeth. In the buccal cavity, saliva present. Saliva is an enzyme present within the salivary gland; saliva is alkaline and contains the enzyme called ptyalin, mixes in food and weakened it into small pieces help its rapid digestion, the digestion of carbohydrate starts from mouth cavity, this enzyme converts a number of the insoluble starches of carbohydrate into soluble sugars or glucose.

CHAPTER 2

Vegetables

The vegetable may be a crucial item of our diet, alkaline, rich in vitamin A, C, and minerals like calcium and iron. Vegetables are the foremost concentrative source of nutrients and enormous variety available everywhere the earth. It's best to eat day to day in several types, and better to eat in raw form. They form roughage in our diet and are best to the obese person does help to manage weight. Vegetables often categorized into a special group: Root and tubers; Radish, carrot, potatoes and turnip, ginger, taro sweet potatoes are included. Green leafy veggies; Broccoli, cabbage, mustard, spinach, fenugreek leaves, kale, coriander, beans, and pea. People who want to reduce weight eat more leafy veggies; the presence of bulk will fill the stomach without having many calories, best for diabetic patients. Dark green leafy veggies have more Vitamins and minerals because of the presence of chlorophyll, more chlorophyll means more vitamin A. 100 grams of green veggies to satisfy the necessity of Vitamin and mineral. Other veggies are tomatoes, bottle guard, asparagus, and each one other veggie. These leaves are low in calories but they form the roughage in our diet and also best for constipate person. Salt of potash combined with vegetable acids helps in maintain the alkaline reserve of the body.

The knowledge of the nutritive value of green leafy vegetables and green tops are essential and it'll go extended because of maintaining a healthy life. It should include in meals especially raw veggies are the only to eat. Winter veggies Radish, carrot, turnip, green beans, cauliflower et al. in these green tops are radishes, carrots, and turnips, in these vegetables have green tops, which usually removed before cooking and thrown away, most of the people do not know that these green tops are edible and for nutritional value, as compare to other root parts that eaten. People have a misconception about using these green tops.

Broccoli

Broccoli green in color, and vegetables a touch like cauliflower, great taste with raw or cooked it contains vitamin B1, B2, B3, B6, iron, magnesium, potassium and zinc, sulfur-containing compound. It's a superb source of vitamin K and C and an honest source of folate it also provides fibers and low in calories. Antioxidant, and protect the body from free radicals. Bitter gourd Dark green in color, Vitamin B, C, phosphorus, protein, zinc, and calcium are in. because of good nutrients best for sugar, Jaundice, paralysis, swelling, and belly fatso.

Bitter gourd

Bottle gourd Bottle ground green in color, bitter in taste, it contains vitamin C, K, calcium, rich in proteins, and omega3 acid. Its seeded oil used to relieve body pain. it's many health benefits; weight loss quickly, will never gain weight; boil 50-gram bottle ground with 2 glass of water until remains 1 glass, drink it daily for 1 month. For headache; 50 gram bulk, mash and apply on the forehead. Cook with the yellow pulse and eat in cough. Its tender leaves and tendrils are edible and contain vitamins and minerals quite fruit. Its peel cooks too and has many benefits; it helps in maintaining a healthy heart and convey down bad cholesterol. Its juice is nice for diabetic patients. it stabilizes the blood sugar level and also maintains blood sugar. It helps to reduce inflammation within the liver and kidneys. It helps in easing the matter related to constipation. Its fiber helps to remain the digestive system active. It helps to treat tract infections.

Beetroot

It is Reddish sweet in taste it contains vitamin A, B, C, H, Glucose, Iron, protein and carbohydrates it's extremely tasty vegetable can cook with meat or alone or mixed with other vegetables like turnip, spinach can cook with or without leaves but better to eat with leaves. Eat with mixed salad dish to remain the body fresh and healthy. Its soup has great taste; make a soup with tomatoes, ginger, garlic, and turnip add salt to taste and ¼ teaspoon black pepper.

Its soup increases red blood cells for people who want to scale back include a salad dish at lunchtime. Cauliflower White in color with small green stem, slightly bit sweet in taste vitamin A, B, E, phosphorus good for kidney and piles patients, Eat with meat, not with potato, gastric, add ginger and ground spicy powder. It's very healthy with great taste. For people who have gastric problems add a little piece of ginger. Chickpea Chickpeas are green in color, sweet in taste. Calcium, vitamin A, B, C, E, H, phosphorus, sulfur, zinc, protein, and carbohydrate are in. Good for liver problems, improve digestion, reduce of risk several diseases, weight loss, high in protein, and excellent replacement of meat. Cabbage's light green and white, purple in color, different colors in several countries too. Vitamin A, B, C, protein, and carbohydrate are in. Eat as a salad, mix with other vegetables, don't eat alone, and add some ginger, don't cook with potatoes, and cook with meat.

Coriander leaves; Green color it contains vitamin K and a little amount of folate, manganese, potassium, and choline, beta carotene, beta-cryptoxanthin, Lutein, and zeaxanthin. Health benefits; it is a fragrant, antioxidant-rich herb. It helps to reduce blood sugar, promote heart, and fight infection, skin, and digestive health. It can easily increase the daily meal.

Eggplant

 Eggplant Purple and white in color-rich in iron, phosphorus, vitamin A, B and C Good for heart, noon constipate but don't eat more.

Tasty cooking method;

 Make paste and eat ½ kg; dig two pieces with stem, boil 1 glass of water, mix 250-gram curd. Add ½ teaspoon garlic past, ½ teaspoon flavored salt to taste, mix well, place a site. In a pan, add 1-tablespoon oil after 1 minute adds ¼-teaspoon cumin until brown add eggplant mixture. Cook for five minutes, sterile, and eat.

Another method; 1 tablespoon red chili powder, ¼ teaspoon turmeric powder, salt to taste, garlic paste 1 tablespoon. White sesame seeds, white cumin, coconut powder, coriander, roast, and crush all, add salt to taste. Mix altogether in a bowl add tamarind water and garlic paste. Fill in ½ kg eggplant (cut into two joint bottoms, within rock bottom of it. Before filling, first place ¼- teaspoon salt within rock bottom of each eggplant. In a separate pan, add 3 tablespoons of oil, add filled eggplant, and cook in 1 glass of water until tender. this is often best for healthy heart and brain function.

Fenugreek leaves; its dark green in color, bitter in taste, a rich source of fiber, proteins, and iron. Nutrition content; in 100g amount: calories = 323 kcal, Carbohydrates = 58% of the daily valve it's documented within the subcontinent is an ancient spice, dried fenugreek leaves used to add flavor and also available in powder form too, its seeds are also comm. in cooking, they yellow amber colored seeds and utilized in pickles but in winter season it's used fresh. Researchers say it, Good for the center, good digestive systems, bone health, prevent anemia, a strong antioxidant, lowering blood sugar levels, boosting testosterone levels, lower inflammation, this a magical herb for diabetic and hear patients.

Cucumber Green full of nutrients, low in calories, high in many important vitamins and minerals. It contains only 16 calories during a cup of cucumber with its peel and without peel 15.4 percent of daily vitamin C, 4 percent of daily potassium, 3 percent daily fiber Benefits; it's antioxidant weight loss and lower blood sugar. Great for a flat stomach, helps the body to relax down. Fresh juice is the best rejuvenation tonic, highly hydrating and alkalizing drink rich in vitamin A, C, K, magnesium, potassium, and silicon.

Corn: Whole corn yellow in color, sweet in taste, and contains high fiber content and valuable Vitamin B12, minerals such as zinc, copper, manganese, and magnesium. Corn is a good source of antioxidants carotenoids, zeaxanthin, and lutein.

Health benefits: high in proteins, Vitamin C, preserve healthy skin, helpful for both mother and baby during pregnancy due to rich in folic acid and contains zeaxanthin and pathogenic which reduce the risk of birth defect in baby and also protect the baby from muscular degeneration and physiological problems. It is soothing constipation due to high fiber content, lower blood sugar, and cholesterol level, and an excellent choice for diabetic and cholesterol patients. Reduce the risk of anemia. Eating plain corn helping with weight loss, the insoluble fiber feeds good bacteria in the gut

Spinach: It is a leafy green vegetable. It is a super-food. It contains Vitamin A, high in Vitamin C and K, fiber, and a great source of iron, calcium, magnesium, and antioxidants.

Health benefits: It is healthy and nutrient-rich food and includes in the daily diet. Study shows that good for diabetic, cancer prevent, asthma, lowering blood pressure, bone health, promote digestive regularity, prevent constipation, healthy skin and hair

Bell pepper

It has several colors such as red, green, and yellow. Tasteless but crunchy, red bell peppers are said to be the sweetest and juiciest, fully ripe, and mature version of green bell pepper then becomes orange and yellow gradually but all are good for health. All bell pepper has vitamin C, but red bell peppers have 1.5 times more vitamin C and 11 times more beta-carotene antioxidants. All peppers color comes from same plant red peppers are most nutrients due to vine longest while green is harvested earlier before to turn yellow, orange and as they become older, changes are made in flavor nutrients qualities. It is good as a pain reliever as ginger does.

Tomato

Ripe red, unripe green in color and sour, loaded with nutrients; Vitamin A, B, C, H, and Iron, best for health, liver, heart, diabetic, digestive system, stomach, teeth, weak children. Do not eat those in cold and cough, and Diphtheria, chest patients. Eat with mixed vegetables or only with onion cannot cook alone but can eat alone without a cook. Its juice also good for health, take 25 litter tomato juice to add ¼ teaspoon black pepper and salt to taste, it will be very tasty and good for blood cells, 1 big size tomato eat in the morning for diabetic patient, kidney swelling, for blood cells and jaundice patients.

It removes skin dryness. Add in every meal dish. It is good for children. It is good for pregnant women, during feeding, for the digestive normal system. Add in salad dish with other vegetables like Radish, turnip, beetroot, and onion.

Taro

Health benefits: It is a root vegetable, rich in fiber and low in calories, contains Vitamin A, C, beta-carotene, cryptoxanthin, copper, manganese, zinc, magnesium, gluten-free, C, E, low in fat and sodium. Good piles patients, Eat with meat not with potato, for gastric, add ginger and ground spicy powder.

 Health benefit: It is anti-cancer properties, control blood sugar, help in losing weight due to very low in calories, reduce your risk of heart disease, reduces fatigue due to low glycemic index, heals acne scars, glowing skin, good for digestion it has a good amount of fiber that is useful for the digestive process. One cup of taro has 0.1g fat and cholesterol which help to prevent hardening of the arteries, It can give 10% of the daily required vitamin E that is essential to prevent the risk of a heart attack, In one cup of taro only 20 mg of sodium that helps to maintain kidney problems due to low in sodium. Vitamin C, 11% in one-cup taro, Vitamin C acts as an antioxidant to remove toxins from your body and detoxifies it, to boost you're immune.

Taro also has a low glycemic index; this helps to break down glucose in the liver slowly and aids in weight loss and lower blood sugar. Taro provides long-lasting energy. It is useful for hypoglycemia, slow down the aging process. To protect against diseases due to Vitamin A, B, C, beta-carotene, cryptoxanthin, copper, manganese, zinc, magnesium, gluten-free, cholesterol-free, and low in sodium.

To protect against diseases and muscle health, protect against cancer it has very high in vitamin A and leaves and roots contain polyphenols, which is great antioxidants. Taro roots have more than seventeen amino acids and omega -3 oils that are essential to main good health; this has omega-3 and six oils which are required for maintaining cardiovascular health, cancer prevention, and other diseases, versatile and easy to add to the diet. Its taste enhances when cooking with meat gravy or spinach.

Green onion

It contains an excellent source of vitamin A, K, C, B6, folate, copper, zinc, magnesium, phosphorus, iron, and potassium.

Health benefits are the combination of onion and green onion, very low in saturated fat, sodium, and cholesterol, antioxidants, and compound that fight inflammation.

Best health benefits due to the best nutrients in. Make the healthiest salad with kale, lettuce, spinach, and other raw vegetables tomatoes, cucumber, cauliflower, and boiled beans. Best skin health, it also removal of dark spot and other blemishes from the skin, bleaching properties are naturally present in lemon help to improve the overall complexion of the skin.

Bauhinia variegate: Flowers, purple, yellow, red and white, a layer is a dark brown, best for women, It's flower and beans, cooks and good for intestine insect, piles patient, motion, blood dysentery.

Kale

Green leafy in color, high in fibers, potassium, calcium, copper, powerful antioxidants, Vitamin A, B6, C, K, and Iron It has health benefits due to best nutrients in. Make the healthiest salad with kale, lettuce, spinach, and other raw vegetables tomatoes, cucumber, cauliflower, and boiled beans.

Lemon

Green and yellow in color, sour in taste, rich in vitamin C, Lemon improves the taste of any meal. Add lemon juice in salad dishes to make it best and digestive. In summer, cut one lemon, make juice add salt to taste and 1 teaspoon sugar for 1 glass water, add a pinch of black pepper and drink, immediately release energy, make you fresh. Best skin health, it also removal of dark spot and other blemishes from the skin, bleaching properties are naturally present in lemon help in improving the overall complexion of the skin.

Drink daily one glass water mix 1 tablespoon lemon juice, within 3 days get a good result.

Lettuce or salary
Green in color, it contains vitamin A, B, C, K, Iron, antioxidant green leaves, low fibers but rich in water, calcium, potassium and folate, magnesium and phosphorus

Health benefits; Eat for a strong body and maintain digestive system, liver, and blood system, Eat a salad with tomato; eat two leaves at a time. Do not eat lettuce alone, you will get sick.

Mint

Dark green in color, vitamin A, B, C, phosphorus, and zinc are in. Its sauce is best for all digestive problems, vomiting, and motion. It's oil also used. Mint used to improve dish quality. Dry mints leave are used in white pulse, potatoes, meat curry, taro root curry, in different mince items and add in daily cooking, its tea is best in vomiting; method to prepare tea; Wash few leaves add 1 glass of water; boil until ½ remains, Lukewarm, drink. It has a natural source of eye health, to keep eyes maintain.

Garlic; garlic contains Vitamin A, C, H, Iron, and zinc, phosphorus, rich in sulfuric acid. It is good for lots of diseases and other treatments due to their chemical properties. Garlic Salsa is best for the digestive system.

method to prepare garlic salsa; garlic paste 1 tablespoon, add 1 tablespoon red chili powder salt to taste, add some water make a paste. In pan heat ¼ cup mustard oil for 10 minutes on a medium-low frame, after 10 minutes, cool until a little warm, add ¼ teaspoon cumin seeds, heat again on the low frame until brown, add chili garlic paste, add ½ glass of water, sterile constantly; cook until water dry, fry for 1 minute.

Another salsa's method; garlic paste ¼ teaspoon, add mint paste 1 bunch, add green coriander paste 2 bunches, add chili powder ½ teaspoon, add green chili paste 1 teaspoon, add cumin powder ¼ teaspoon, add dry pomegranate seeds paste, add salt to taste. Add them together, mix well, and eat with any meal, very tasty and digestive.

Ginger

In ginger, a compound called gingerol, pain reliever. For health Dry ginger powder is used for a lot of treatment, For the digestive system, cough, vomiting, flu, cough, stomach pain, gastric problems, ginger may prevent diabetic kidney damage. It is help in nausea and morning sickness. it's tea best in cough, high in calories, high in sugar but ginger has a very long history of use in forms of alternative medicine, it helps in digestion, flu, and common cold and reduce nausea, can be used fresh, dried powder form, oil and juice and sometimes added to processed foods and cosmetics. It can treat morning sickness, may reduce muscle pain, soreness, reducing symptoms of osteoarthritis.

It is help in digestion and another stomach discomfort.

Ginger powder may reduce menstrual pain, lower cholesterol levels, protect against Alzheimer's disease and improve brain function and a substance found in raw ginger also help in cancer as research showed but not in all cancer.

Onion

It is mostly used to make curry with meat. Do not eat at night. Eat onion in a salad or only with a tortilla in the daytime. Common benefits of onion; Good for diarrhea, add with apple cider, patient eat. Apply onion paste on white hair, black hair will be grown. Apply onion juice to a black spot on the body, which will be disappeared. Take 2 drops of onion juice, drop into the nose, nose bleeding will be stopped. Eat Onion without a cook, keep with you, will never suffer from dangerous diseases. In summer, the smell of onion affected a person by heatstroke. Urinary infection one small onion boil in 1-liter water until remains 1 small glass, drink patient, Eruption patient, drink boil onion water, boil onion(peeled) 1 add 3 cup water until remains 1 cup, cool and drink.

Red and green chili

 Spicy, it contains Vitamin A, C, zinc, iron, phosphorus, protein. Boost the immune system. best for all body organs, diarrhea medical researcher says, In 100-gram chili includes 100-gram Vitamin C, Vitamin C is essential for blood circulation; it is best for healing, blood pressure and many teeth problems, onion pickle is also for a healthy body, add in meal list.

Garlic

Chemical properties; vitamin A, C, H, Iron, and zinc, phosphorus, rich in sulfuric acid, Good for lots of diseases and other treatment due to its chemical properties. Garlic Salsa is best for the digestive system, can eat with lentil, vegetable, or even meat, very tasty.

Method:

Garlic paste 1 tablespoon, add 1-tablespoon red chili powder salt to taste, add some water make a paste.

In pan heat ¼ cup mustard oil for 10 minutes on a medium-low frame, after 10 minutes, cool until a little warm, add ¼ teaspoon cumin seeds, heat again on the low frame until brown, add chili garlic paste, add ½ glass of water, sterile constantly; cook until water dry, fry for 1 minute.

Another salsa's method:

Garlic paste ¼ teaspoon, add mint paste 1 bunch, add green coriander paste 2 bunches, add chili powder ½ teaspoon, add green chili paste 1 teaspoon, add cumin powder ¼ teaspoon, add dry pomegranate seeds paste, add salt to taste. Add them together, mix well, and eat with any meal, very tasty and digestive.

Coriander leaves

Green in color It contains vitamin K and a small amount of folate, manganese, potassium, and choline, beta carotene, beta-cryptoxanthin, Lutein, and zeaxanthin. Health benefits; It is a fragrant, antioxidant-rich herb. It helps to reduce blood sugar, promote heart, and fight infection, skin, and digestive health. It can easily add to the daily meal.

Mushroom

Mushrooms contain fiber, copper, potassium, magnesium, and zinc, rich in vitamins B such as riboflavin, B1, B2 folate, B3, and minerals. It is also low in calories and fat, free of cholesterol, In other words, can say mushrooms are packed with nutritional value, vitamins help the body to get energy from food and help to form red blood cells and vitamin B for the importance of the healthy brain. 1 cup of mushroom contains 15 calories and only 2.3 grams of carbohydrates.

Lime

It contains vitamin C, anti-oxidants, anti-inflammation, a good source of magnesium, potassium. Health benefits are to reduce heart disease; lowers blood sugar, improve digestion system, weight loss and fight against infection

Loquat

Yellow in color, it contains carbohydrates, proteins, vitamin A, B6, C, calcium, iron, potassium, magnesium, sodium, and dietary fibers. It is health benefits due to its nutrients value.

Radish

It is white, red, and sweet and bitter in taste. Vitamin C, phosphorus, iron, and calcium are in. good for jaundice and liver problems. Eat as salad also good with meat; its leaves are also good to eat. Best for kidney stone patient; eat daily stone will removed in form of sand. Best for pile patients, abstract radish leaves, add some sugar, drink patient. For any liver problem, 1 radish, keep under open-air overnight,   eat in the morning, a patient will be recovered soon. For urine problems, eat 1 radish daily. Radish pickle good for piles, pancreas, all urine problems. Radish eats with chili powder for teeth and gum patient's teeth will be strong.

Make radish pickle with apple cider for the best result in all liver problems. For asthma patients, add salt and honey, eat the patient daily. For an irregular digestive patient, eat Radish with salt and warm water. For kin allergy; Onion juice 1 tablespoon, rub on allergy places with a fingertip.

Sponge ground

It is green in color, tasteless, Rich in water, vitamin C, K, calcium glucose, good vegetable for all digestive problems.

Moringa

The complete tree is good for health, the bean is green in color It contains Vitamin A, B, C, E, H, calcium, zinc Its bean, flowers and leaves good for health, bean and flowers cook with meat, mince, and yellow pulse. It is best for stomach pain, and cough. Its pickle is best for back pain, joint pain, and gastric problems. It is also best for kidney stones and sand. Do not eat during angry. It is good for paralyze, joints diseases. It helps to keep eyesight fast.

Tamarind

Dark brown but unripe green in color, sore in taste, it is rich in nutrients Vitamin B1, B3, the polyphenols antioxidant and anti-inflammatory, mineral and Vitamin C

Amazing health benefits;

Tamarind, a complete plant is used for treatment, such as seed, layer, paste, root, leaves, and juice. (I'll write it's a complete method to use in another book but few benefits are protected against heart disease, diabetes, and cancer, its seeds extract may also help in lower blood pressure. Pulp extract help in lose body weight but chronic kidney patient avoid to eat it due to potassium in.

Tamarind juice adds in vegetables, pulses, curry and can drink juice with a pinch of salt and red chili powder. Tamarind paste 25 grams boil with 2 cups of water brings it to boil, cover, strain, and drink lukewarm, good for the digestive process.

Chickpea

Chickpeas are green in color, sweet in taste, Nutrient value; Calcium, vitamin A, B, C, E, H, phosphorus, sulfur, zinc, protein, carbohydrate **Benefits**; good for liver problems, improve digestion, reduce of risk several diseases, weight loss, high in protein and excellent replacement of meat.

Eggplant

Purple and white in color, rich in iron, phosphorus, vitamin A, B, and C, good for heart, noon constipate but do not eat more.

A method to make a delicious dish;

Take ½ kg cut into two pieces with stem, boil 1 glass of water, mix 250-gram curd. Add ½-teaspoon garlic paste, ½-teaspoon chili powder, salt to taste, mix well, place a site. In a pan add 1 tablespoon oil after 1 minute adds ¼ teaspoon cumin seed until brown add eggplant mixture.

Cook for 5 minutes, sterile, and eat.

Another Method

1- Teaspoon chili powder, ¼-teaspoon turmeric powder, salt to taste, garlic paste 1 tablespoon. White sesame seeds, white cumin seed, coconut powder, coriander, roast and crush all, add salt to taste. Mix in a bowl with tamarind water and garlic paste, fill in ½ kg eggplant (cut into two joint bottoms, in the bottom of it, before filling, first place ¼ teaspoon salt in the bottom of each eggplant. In a separate pan, add 3 tablespoons of oil, add filled eggplant, and cook in 1 glass of water until tender. This is best for healthy heart and brain function.

Aloe Vera

The surface is green in color but the gel is colorless contains Vitamin C, E, zinc Health benefits; these vegetables are also best for treatment; help in swelling, stomach pain, any sort of body burn, sunburn, gum and teeth surgery, insect bites, any sort of mouth infection, for healing. Aloe Vera used in shampoo, powder, cream, lotion, body lotion, Shaving gel, gel, and for face skin and wrinkles. Other vegetables like celery, leeks, artichokes, squash, zucchini, lettuce, mushrooms, Brussels sprouts are also healthy vegetables.

CHAPTER 3

Fruits

Fruit consuming regularly to help in digestion, boosting the immune system, manage high blood pressure, promoting blood circulation, balance in cholesterol level and diabetes, preventing the risk of cancer, support in respiratory health and cardiovascular system, treating inflammation, and strengthen bones. Fruits contain minerals, salts, and carbohydrates such as laevulose and fructose. Citric fruits are a good source of Vitamin C such as oranges, guava. Papaya and mangoes are rich in Vitamin A. When eating certain fruits with skin contain cellulose and assists in normal bowel movement. Green fruits to help indigestion for example green papaya and green bananas.

Apple

It is red, yellow and green. Sweet and sore in a test, it contains Vitamin C, a lot of iron, calcium, and phosphorous, low sugar fruit, high in fiber and antioxidant.

Benefits of apple;

Apple is best for remarkable health, superb for healthy brain, liver, kidney, function; it improves memory, makes blood cells, Strong brain function, relieve in headache, best for skin care, help in stomach pain, for intestine, dysentery, for cough and thirsty feelings. It's a perfect snack between meals if anyone feels hungry.

Apricot

It is light yellow in color and unripe green in color, sweet in taste, and sore unripe. It contains vitamin A, C, E, carotenoids (lutein and zeaxanthin), beta-carotene, a small number of calories and carbohydrates in one apricot, a good source of fibers, low calories.
It protects the eyes from damage, good for diabetes and weight loss, excellent to protect the heart from free radical damages, and lowers blood pressure by relaxing blood arteries and vessels. It has enough amounts of soluble and insoluble fibers but high in soluble fibers. One cup of fresh apricot has 74 calories and 14.5 grams of sugar naturally. Dried apricot contains 78 calories and 17 grams of sugar. This fruit is eating as a whole. Do not eat too much in dried form, it can create health issues due to more sugar and weight gain too.

Banana

Banana (peeled), off-white but the skin is yellow and green, sweet in taste, it includes vitamin A, B6, and E and essential minerals. The benefits of banana; it has lots of health benefits including weight maintains, good for the trough, and cough, complete bananas are good for human's health. Intestine problems, Constipation, Tong sore, Urine disorder, dysentery and motion, heart problems, strong brain function, for cold, cough, and fever.

Berries

 All berries are the same in nutritional value, a most powerful source of antioxidants, good for all healthy brain functions and other body organs, can eat alone or mix with other fruit; blackberries are one of the best fruit after apple.

Coconut

It contains high nutrients and rich in vitamin C, E, B1, B3, B5, B6, and minerals, loaded with fiber and powerful fatty acids called medium-chain triglycerides, white in color, best for tired, sleep and release energy.
Healthy benefits; it digestive, heart health, weight loss

Custard Apple

It is greenish-black in color, sweet taste and a good smell of very soft white inner side seeds cover with pulp. It has vitamin C, antioxidants, high in potassium, magnesium
 Health benefits; Protect the heart from cardiac disease, control blood pressure, best for weight gain; eat daily two, after a few days weight, will be increased. Best for dry skin problems, high blood pressure, kidney problems, liver, stomach acidity, intestine problem, dysentery, and cough.

Dates

Dates are good health and glowing skin, dark brown, It contains phosphorous, calcium, protein, carbohydrates, zinc, and fats, Dates are best on this planet; it called happy fruit due to its benefits.
Health benefits; Antioxidants, a good source of vitamins and minerals, can be blood sugar balance, good for blood pressure, help to maintain bone mass, good in dried and fresh.

High healthy fruit add to a daily meal list

Mal berry

is also a small berry, purple in color, a taste of it is incredible which has a combination of sour, bitter and acidic, the texture is similar to grapes due to the presence of a white color pulp inside. This fruit has great nutritional value and health benefits. It contains carbohydrates, proteins, calcium, phosphorus, iron and dietary fiber, sodium, vitamin A, B1, B2, B3, C, low glycemic index (low glycemic is control blood glucose metabolism.

Health benefits are;

Source of antioxidants, source of sodium (increase the performance of a nervous system and need for blood regulation, in the presence of vitamin A, to promote good vision and prevents macular degeneration, promoting blood cells and the body metabolism.
Vitamin B1, B2, and B6 found in it; helps to maintain the heart and nerve function, deficiency of this vitamin may lead to certain health problems including anorexia, muscle weakness, and nerve damages. Its barks are used for the treatment of rheumatism (swelling of joints), for respiratory problems (asthma, colds, bronchitis), drink juice;
mulberry juice, add ¼ teaspoons ginger in 1 glass of mal berry juice or can add ¼ lemon juice instead of ginger juice and drink.

Drink 1 glass of its juice daily to avoid:
Muscle problems and bones problems (proteins and potassium are responsible to strengthen the muscle and good muscle and build healthy bones in the presence of calcium, fibers; to prevent stomachache, nausea and any other digestive problems such as diarrhea, control blood pressure and soothing the liver, to prevent stroke, help to prevent diabetes. Lower the cancer risk; breast and liver cancer, to treat anemia and prevent chronic fatigue. To help in healing wounds and eczema; grind the leaves and apply them on the skin, leave for a few minutes to let them work. To prevents the free radicals. It is an antioxidant and anti-inflammation.

Grapes

Light green, red, white, and black when dry called currants (dry grapes), sweet and sour, Vitamin A, C, calcium, protein, carbohydrates, manganese are in and glucose and antioxidants
Benefits; It is filled with vitamin C and antioxidants can help to revitalize skin, protect from ultraviolet radiation and free radicals cause, wrinkles, dark spots, and cancer, for gain weight eat lot and motion, 2 gram best in motion, good for brain, heart, liver, lungs, and intestine, make red blood cell, good in cold, cough, scrofula and influenza

Grapefruit

Orange in color, it is rich in vitamin C, fiber, antioxidants, and helps in lower cholesterol.

Health benefits;

This fruit best to reduce weight. Keeps low cholesterol level in the blood. Eat daily to keep weight control, there is no specific method to eat this fruit but eat a whole with fiber because fiber eats fat so the weight will never be increased when drinking its juice add a pinch black salt and pepper, drink a glass of grapefruit to burn belly fat. Grapefruit has full of soluble fiber called pectin, high cholesterol patients eat as a whole daily in the morning to control cholesterol level within six months.

Guava

It is green in color and red, good taste and smell. It is rich in vitamin A, C, phosphorus, calcium, and iron. Good for stomach, nose bleed, irregular period, piles, heart, and digestive system, eat before the meal, after meal it does constipate, beast for brain functions. The seed is not eatable but can kill the abdominal insect, do not eat more seeds.

Jambolan

It is purple in color, bitter in taste. Rich in iron, a good level of vitamin A-C
Health benefits; Jambolan is best for stomach, liver, pancreas, and kidney functions. The complete tree is the best of the best, pulp, leaves, fruits, seeds. It keeps skin fresh and healthy.

Make its seed powder,

1-teaspoon powder mix with 2- teaspoon milk
Make paste apply on the skin to reduce acne.

 Amazing health benefits;

Jambolan is extremely good for diabetes person.
 it has low glycemic index, which ensures conversion of
sugar and starch to energy, reducing the blood levels,
good for eyes, its fruits, seeds, leaves, and bard, all are
good in a different way, its seeds, when taken with
yogurt, helps in breaking kidney stones; bark and seed
powder helps in gastric disorder treatment such as
indigestion ad diarrhea. Superb natural blood purifier
ensuring oxygenated blood supplier. Its juice is good
for increasing memory levels and, with anemia,
respiratory disorders like asthma, also good for teeth
and gums. For full enjoy it, black salt, sprinkle over it,
and eat. Patients undergoing surgery must avoid eating
Jambolan as it might lead to low blood sugar levels. Do
not on an empty stomach. Consumption of milk
avoided one hour before and after eating this fruit.

Litchi

Red in color, It contains a good amount of antioxidant,
Vitamin C, B complex and a decent source of copper
and fibers

Health benefits; In the presence of the rich source of
nutrients that is required for the production of blood
cells, the presence of fibers helps to keep weight
maintain. Good fiber and vitamin B complex increase

metabolism, carbohydrate, fat, protein, good for heart health, help o prevent diseases. Protect the skin cells. Eat litchi several times a week, help to relieve the kidney pain due to kidney stones. Increase immune system

Loquat

Orange fleshed in color, sweet, and citron in taste; research shows that this fruit's extract contains antioxidants, low in calories, and an excellent source of vitamin A, B, potassium, manganese, magnesium, and fibers.

Health benefits; This fruit is best for a strong immune system, inflammation, diabetes, aging pain, bacterial infection, cancer, allergy, and other health issues.

Mulberry

Reddish pink in color, sweet in taste, Vitamin A, C, D, Iodine, potassium, copper, calcium, zinc, glucose, fats, phosphorus, niacin, and iron.

Health benefits; It has lots of health benefits which are related to the nutrients present in it, easily digest within 2 hours. Full of nutrients in 250 grams, eat 20 to 30 gram daily, a patient will recover from diphtheria. Best for healthy brain function, tired, angry persons, belly fat and cold and cough patient drink its cold juice daily in the morning.

Mango

Mango is called the king of fruits; it has good flavor and smell, sweet in taste, rich in phosphorous, magnesium, calcium, iron, potassium, zinc, carbohydrates, and proteins Mango has 25% glucose and 75% clean water.

Mango is best for the Liver, chest, heart, brain, lungs, and stomach provide energy to all these organs of our body, do not eat empty stomach due to acidity, makes blood cells. Complete mango plant is superb for the human being.

Benefits of mango leaves

Pluck the first flower from the mango tree and rub it on your hand, it will remain in your hand the whole year, whenever any insect bites on anyone's hand or in your hand rub on that place. For Eyes infection or miner eyes problems; for effected eyes, such as aches, swelling, eye infection and water falling and week eyesight for long-distance

Method to use;

Mango fresh leaves 1kg, crush wet in a copper pot add eight-letter of water. Place overnight, in the morning cook it until half kg water remains, stain, again cook make a thick paste, keep in a neat bottle when required, take one drop to add one tables spoon of mineral water and take one or two drops into effected eyes, three times a day.

Melon

It is yellow with a green strip, rich in vitamin D, and calcium, potassium, glucose, phosphorus, vitamin A and B zinc, and carotene.

Health benefits; best for kidney stone and jaundice patients, there is no specific method to eat, ½ or full melon, eat daily, if eating as a patient, also can eat as fruit mix dish for health. It helps to gain weight gain.

Papaya

It is rich sources of antioxidant nutrients such as carotenoids can neutralize free radicals vitamin A, B, C and also proteins, carbohydrates, enzymes, potassium, copper, magnesium, and fibers

Benefits

It is good for diabetic patients.
It has used in traditional remedies in many ailments; the juice for cancers, tumors, warts, and corns, and skin thickness, can promote oxidative stress, which is lead to disease, antioxidants, can neutralize free radicals. The roots and extract, use for cancers of the uterus, syphilis, hemorrhoids, tropical infection, and to remove mineral concretions in the urine. Unripe fruit, as a mild laxative and can promote oxidative stress, which leads to disease.
Good for weight loss eat daily after a meal, best for cough, gastric problems. Eat as a fruit mix dish. Full ripe papaya cab is used for immediately cooking meat.

Apply papaya bulk mix with salt and pepper as required; apply on meat pieces, left for 20 minutes, and cook. Do not cook in a pressure cooker; cook in the pan under steam for 10 to 15 minutes.

Peach

Peach has beautiful in color is good for summer hot weather, soft, fleshy stone and juicy, sweet and sore, it is packed with nutrients and antioxidants; peach has protein, vitamin A, C, carbohydrate, calcium, phosphorus, Iron. Fibers are present and very low calories good for all body organs such as heart, liver, kidney, stomach, diabetes. A powerful full antioxidant that helps maintains the immune system and weight loss due to low calories. Protect skin. It helps to improve digestion. Avoid allergy symptoms. The dietary specialist said; do not eat too many per day. Overeating can create side effects such as heartburn, diarrhea, and bloating.

Pear

It is green in color; rich in Vitamins

Health benefits;

It is good for the acidic patient, piles, dry skin, any liver diseases, blood pressure, and heart diseases patient are regularly eat, these organ will not create problems again.

Pineapple

It is light yellow, sweet, and sore in taste, it is rich in vitamin A, C, carbohydrates, calcium, potassium, and proteins. Best in hot summer weather, drink its juice, peel, takeout seeds, and crush, make juice add ice and drink, best for kidney problems, liver and stomach. Make pineapple's paste, peel 1 pineapple, boil with ½ glass of water add some brown sugar, cook until a thick paste, this is best for heart and kidney.

Pomegranate

It is reddish-brown or red in color, sweet and sore in taste but sometimes very sweet. It is rich in tannin, carbohydrates, fat, protein, Vitamins, minerals nitric, and citric acids.

For health, it is best as a fruit as well as traditional treatment, help in erosive gastritis, enteritis, reflux esophagitis, irritating bowel disorder. Increase blood red cell, it has vitamin C which is best for skin problems like allergy, increases eyesight, pain killer, eats sweet pomegranate always. Increase hair growth and weight control digestive system, its juice best for heart and liver, can drink during vomiting and motion. Sweet pomegranate is good for cough and throat infection. The complete plant used for body treatment.

Quince

Quince is yellow; it contains copper, Sodium, potassium, iron, vitamin C magnesium

Healthy properties

Person can feel the burden of the heart, relaxes the heart and releases the tightness from the chest. If pregnant women drink, to remove heart issues and keep babies healthy, it cures many heart problems, control LDL (LDL are the lipid harmful as they clog the artery and cause an obstruction), while HDL well it lowing LDL and high HDL. Relaxes the heart and releases the tightness. Vitamin C, which helps to control the immune system well. It is cancer prevents and weight loss abilities.

Sapodilla

Its color brown, sandy, round and oval shape, evergreen tree, sweet in taste, contains dietary fiber, vitamin A, B, and C also antioxidants.

Health benefits;

Fresh is a good source of minerals like copper, iron, potassium, and vitamin niacin, folate, and pantothenic acid. It composes of soft, easily digestive pulp made of simple sugars like fructose and sucrose.

Unripe fruits possess white, hard, inedible pulp that secretes sticky latex-containing toxic substance saponin, milky latex gradually disappears and white flesh turns brown as the fruit ripe. Ripen becomes soft, sweet taste and smooth or grainy texture with slight musky flavor, contain about two to 4 or sometimes 10 black, smooth, shiny bean or biconvex shaped, inedible seeds, located at its center. It is a high calories fruit, 100g provides 83 calories, an excellent source of dietary fiber, which makes it a good bulk laxative; this fiber content helps relieve constipation episodes and helps protect the mucosa of the colon from cancer-causing toxins.

Antioxidant rich in polyphenolic compound tannin, research studies suggest that tannins possess astringent properties and shown to have potential anti-inflammatory, antibacterial, anti-parasitic, antiviral effects. The anti-inflammatory effect of tannins helps erosive gastritis, reflux esophagitis, enteritis, and irritating bowel disorders. It has Vitamin C (antioxidant Vitamin), helps the body develop resistance to combat infectious agents, and help scavenge harmful free radicals from the human body) and vitamin A (essential for vision and protection from lung and oral cavity cancers), can maintain healthy skin and mucosa.

Sugarcane

Sweet syrup extracts from bark; are rich in vitamin A, B, C, calcium, iron, and phosphorus. Good for gum and teeth, Stomach patient, kidney stone, student and hard workers, healthy brain function and heart patient

Watermelon

Surface dark green in color; It is full of healthy water but does not drink water after eating. It contains vitamin B 6, thiamine, folate, niacin, potassium, phosphorus, riboflavin, zinc, manganese, selenium, choline, thiamine, and lycopene. Presence of Lycopene; turn foods red and naturally occurs in food that reacts with the human body to trigger the healthy reaction. Helps hydrates, lower inflammation, and oxidative stress, relieve muscle soreness, best for blood pressure, weight loss, asthma, heart health, hydration for the skin, kidney health, and pregnancy, helps the liver process.

All vegetables are important either in root class like potato, carrot, turnip, and radish. all green leafy such as broccoli, cabbage, spinach, mustard, fenugreek leaves, coriander leaves, beans, peas, peppermint and others like tomatoes, bottle gourd, cucumber, and some others.

Winter vegetables such as turnip, radish, carrot all have green tops are edible, and have far more nutritional value than the other root vegetables. Green tops are more nutritious than the actual vegetable.

Fibers

The skin of fruits cover with seeds and the structural parts of edible plants call fibers. Fiber known as roughage and are found in two types: **water-soluble** and **water-insoluble** Fiber.

Soluble fiber

Soluble fiber dissolves in water. Help to control blood sugar levels and reduce cholesterol.

Good sources are barley, oatmeal, beans, nuts, and fruits such as apple, pear, berries, and citrus fruits and **there is no fiber in meat, dairy product, sugar, and refined flour items and most of the fibers remove such as white rice, white bread pastries have had all or most of their fiber removed.**

 Water Insoluble fiber does not dissolve in water;

This is present in whole grains, wheat cereals, carrots, tomatoes, and celery. this type of fiber present in the form of bulk useful in the elimination of intestinal waste, keeping the digestive system clean and healthy, easing bowel movements by bulking up stools and making them easier to pass and flushing cholesterol and harmful carcinogens out of the body.

and also helps to prevent constipation, diarrhea and reduce the risk of gallstones, kidney stone and hemorrhoids A diet high in insoluble fiber from cereals can lower risk for type 2 diabetes and soluble fiber can slow absorption of sugar and improve blood sugar levels of diabetic patients. Many foods contain both soluble and insoluble fiber. The higher fiber is found in natural and unprocessed food. Flaxseeds are small brown seeds high in fibers and omega-3 fatty acids, which can lower blood cholesterol. Many studies suggest that eating food high in fiber can boost the immune system and overall health benefits, losing weight, and maintain a healthy weight. Fiber bulk can help fill full sooner, fiber stays in the stomach longer, helping to eat less, high fibers fruits and vegetables are low in calories so by adding fiber in diet easier to cut calories and maintain weight. Plenty of salad consumed to avoid constipation. The best way to start a meal with a fresh raw salad dish; thoroughly wash all vegetables before cutting, a good salad dish contains minerals and Vitamins.

Seeds, Nuts, and Pulses

Seeds

Chia seeds

Chia seeds are edible seeds and best for health, most nutrient foods around the world it contains large amounts of omega-3 fatty acids, antioxidants, iron, fiber, and significant magnesium, manganese, calcium, and proteins. Omega 3 fatty acids are important for heart and mental health.

Also, maintain insulin levels in the blood and help to weight loss. It used with many types of syrup, juices, and eats to mix in yogurt and oatmeal. The method is to soak before add in any dish or syrup because it will be slightly sick in size and looks nice otherwise; it is too small in dry form.

Flaxseed

Flaxseeds are also important as chia seeds. It contains omega 3 fatty acids, high in proteins, fibers, calcium, iron good for heart health, blood pressure, may reduce risk of cancer, can add all type of foods like the oatmeal, waffle

Aniseeds

Aniseed 1 tablespoon, add 1 pinch of carom seeds, boil for 3 minutes, strain, add mint's powder ½ teaspoon, drink, immediately relieve pain.

Sesame seeds White brown and black contain omega fatty acid, antioxidants, anti-inflammatory properties, fiber, minerals, and a high source of unsaturated fats.

Health benefits:

These seeds are essential for hair growth.

 Anti-aging, wonderful for skin health, healing redness, oil of it boot oral health and remove dental plaque, black sesame seeds help to cure constipation due to high fiber content, boost digestion; the oil found in the seed can lubricate intestine while the fiber helps in smooth bowel movements, a good source of energy due to high-fat content as export says. Rich in magnesium that helps prevent hypertension. Polyunsaturated fats and compound sesame present in it to keep blood pressure levels control. Keeps bone strong. Help fight stress and depression

Fenugreek seeds: It's Contains Vitamin A, C, and D, minerals, and fibers, low in cholesterol, lots of health benefits: Reduce appetite, fat, menstrual cramps, and fever; soothe muscles pain and upset stomach and digestive problems; balance cholesterol and lowering blood sugar.

Black seeds: Black, it is containing Vitamin A, B6, C, D, protein, fat, carbohydrates, fiber, fixed oil, volatile oil, alkaline, mineral, and unlimited health benefits. **I have written all seeds benefit in detail, next book Home remedies.**

Nuts

Nuts and seeds: Nuts are a great source of fibers, a good source of fiber nuts are Almond, Pecans, Walnuts, Pistachios, and Cashews these nuts have more fibers than other nuts, and also a good source of proteins, healthy fats Vitamins, and minerals. Nuts and seeds regulate body weight as their fats are not fully absorbed, they regulate food intake and help burn Nuts and seeds contain unsaturated fats and other nutrients that protective effects against heart disease.

Pulses and beans

Pulses are also useful in the diet because they are rich in protein and cheaper meat and also contain mineral such as iron, calcium, Eat most in a week 1 cup of wheat cooked in milk eat with 1 banana in the morning. 1-cup raw vegetables and ½ cup fried vegetables

½ cup cooked bean or lentil

Whole grain, whole grain bread,

 a small piece of potato or sweet potato

1 cup mixed chopped fruits and a small piece of fruit,

1 cup low-fat milk, non-fat curd, eat in a small amount within a week,

Ice cream or butter, fruit juice, and bar, fried, canned, cream sauce, butter vegetables, white rice, dried fruits, white bread, chips, crackers, cookies, cake, muffins, cold cereal, and cold flavored oatmeal.

Eating like fruits, whole grains or high cereal fiber varieties, vegetables and legumes, beans, fat-free or low-fat dairy, proteins foods seafood, lean meats, eggs. Best foods around the world, are black beans, barriers especially blueberry, spinach, walnuts, avocado, garlic, dark chocolates, and beets due to essential vitamin and minerals, which is required the human body to stay functioning at its best. Our energy requirements change with the type of activity performed by the body and also depend on the age, sex, and weight of a person. Wheat is a staple food all around the world. It contains 70 % starch, 8 to 12% gluten, and 15% water. In whole wheat 1.5 gm fat/100 gm, 11.8 gm protein/100 gm, 1.2 gm fiber/100 gm, calcium .050 gm/100 gm, iron 5.3 mg in 100 gm. Pulses are rich in proteins; it contains 20 to 25% protein, in fact, more protein than other protein foods like fish, egg, meat and other. Pulses are rich in calcium, iron, and lysine. Green leafy vegetables should always be included daily as food export says.

Kidney Beans

A well-balanced diet is essential to maintain a good digestive system it contains all of the nutrients (carbohydrates, fats, proteins, vitamins, and minerals).

According to the body requirement when these components are in proper proportion contribute and satisfy a person's nutritional requirement, it becomes a nutritionally balanced diet. Nutrition impacts health eat well balance diet to live a long and healthy life to provide energy to keep the body in good working condition. Meal of fish or meat, salad, Boiled chickpeas add salad in keeps you healthy also can add some olive oil, the fruit is better than a snack of **popcorn with butter and pizza** or other oily snakes. A balanced diet is to delay the effects of aging as most people remain conscious about it. Foods like berries, avocados, nuts, tomatoes, fish, and minerals all contain certain vitamins that are good for the skin. Berries are full of antioxidants and vitamins, tomatoes contain vitamins C which helps build collagen, making your skin fresh and firmer, slow aging effects eating them promotes cell regeneration for new skin.

Eat plenty of all color fruits contain Vitamin C, all veggies and fruits greater variety, avoid potatoes and French fries, and avoid trans- fat. Peanut butter is high in healthy fats, 100 grams = 588 calories, high in calories content, pure peanut butter, or whole peanut is fine on weight loss diet. Some meals in the daily healthy eating plate will help to control weight. Vegetable juice or soup It is essential for health to make a chart of good eating. Soybean is the richest source of protein; dry soybean oil is an oil of superior quality.

Healthy breakfast

Start your day with a healthy breakfast that keeps your body slim. Healthy breakfast means a breakfast includes protein and healthy fat, keep you fit whole day, no oily food, full of nutrients, carbohydrate, fat, protein and Vitamin, eggs are good and most nutritious foods, previously it is demonized due to high cholesterol but new research shows that eggs are perfectly healthy and safe.

Whatever eating in breakfast but balanced as a food specialist says, and a balanced diet is essential for everyone's health. Whole grain cereals to boost fiber intake at morning time, replace white bread, white rice and pasta to brown bread, brown rice and whole-grain, barley, whole-wheat pasta, bulgur, toast, and sandwiches theses are high in fiber and good in taste, in-home baking use whole grain flour do not use yeast let the dough rise longer. Flaxseeds grind and add to brown bread or other breakfast cereals, sauces, and yogurt. A balanced diet can keep to person look young and delay the effects of aging. Foods like berries, avocados, nuts, tomatoes, fish, and minerals all contain certain vitamins that are good for the skin. Berries are full of antioxidants and vitamins, tomatoes contain vitamins C which helps build collagen, making your skin fresh and firmer, slow aging effects eating them promotes cell regeneration for new skin.

Iron deficiency may cause fatigue, low energy, and irritability. Spinach rich in iron other foods like dark green leafy, seafood, poultry, peas are also rich in iron and best to consume vitamin C, peppers, broccoli and meals are full of vitamin C and iron, antioxidants are spinach, avocados, and yellow corn.

Bananas boost energy, cherry calm nerves, strawberries fight aging, graphs relax blood vessels, and broccoli, pomegranates, avocados, and coconut oil is balancing hormones. The World Healthy lifestyle is a way of living without seriously ill or dying early or mental, physical, and social well-being not merely the absence of disease. Scientific studies have identified those certain types of behavior that contribute to the development of non-communicable diseases and early death.

Knowledge of balance diet is essential from an early age of a child to change of behaviors with family and other related peoples, eggs also takeout from depress an anxiety situation, fruits, whole grain, vegetables, fish, and olive oil help improve the blood vessels and reduce the risk of memory damage.

Fishes are high in omega -3 fatty acids, which is linked to lower levels of beta-amyloid proteins in the blood and improve better vascular health.

Make a weekly mediterranean menu to add your choice of food and needs from Monday to Sunday.

Good nutrition will remain control blood pressure, bad cholesterol, and the immune system. Good nutrition diet including yogurt, oats, tomatoes, black beans, radish, walnuts, carrots, cucumber, and blueberries, pomegranate, grapefruits, strawberries, blackberries, oranges, lentils, and limes. There is some healthiest drink like coffee, green tea, low calories beer, milk, water, fruit juices, best low calories energy drinks, best green juices, you can get all from Amazon. You can prepare some green vegetable juice at home too. Apple cider vinegar is also a good weight loose drink and also improves body skin and remains glowing and healthy. Kid, do not know about healthy, food, and skin glowing.

Meat

Do not avoid meat are also essential for our requirement it is rich in proteins, it consists of muscle fibers held together by connective tissue. Proteins of meats are myosin, muscle albumin and hemoglobin also contain minerals, a certain amount of fat and Vitamin B complex, and a small amount of Vitamin A and C. Younger animal meat will take less time for cooking. Meat should be firm and elastic, with little or no odor. It should not be pale pink color; it is a sign of disease and deep purple color indicate that the animal has not killed fresh.

Mutton is easily digested as compared to meat due to its shorter fibers and tendered but should be a fatless or small amount of fat. In a goat, the flesh is tendered and less fat, and more easily digest.

 The flesh of ducks is darker and not suitable for the stomach. The flesh of partridge is white but tender and delicate fiber, good flavor, and also easy to digest. The flesh of birds has less fat and delicate and largely eaten due to softness.

Organ meats: There are several types of organ meats such as liver, heart, brain, tripe, tongue, and kidney. Organ meat are super food as says export,

they are very high in Vitamin and nutrients,

Vitamin A, B, D, E, K, iron, magnesium, copper and phosphorus, and folate makes beneficially for fertility and for helping avoid fetal defects in a baby heart problems and spine Bifida and presence of Vitamin B6 can help morning sickness but in all organ, meat liver is first because it is so densely packed with nutrients as medical sources say.

Liver

The liver is a nutritional powerhouse and it is the most nutrient-dense food packed with essential nutrients. Some people do not like it as compared to muscle meats; maybe they do not its nutrient value. The liver is rich in Vitamin A and B2 and B9, C, and D also in.

Lever also rich in high-quality protein low in calories and packed with essential minerals, it is easily digested it has contained valuable minerals, and good for anemic patients. A small amount of liver provides 100% of RDI for many essential nutrients; most liver sources are cow, chicken, duck, pig, lamb, and buffalo. The liver has fewer calories than any other meat.

The liver can eat as pan-fried with onion and spices. Beef liver is extremely nutritious and contains a good range of minerals. The liver is in short can say a great source of high-quality protein and this sort of protein intake has been shown to increase metabolic rate, help built muscle, reduce appetite and preserve muscle during weight loss. The liver has fewer calories than other meats.

Tongue: Tongue meat is good for pregnant women and those persons recovering from illness. It is rich in Vitamin B12, calories, fatty acids, choline, zinc, and iron.

Brain: Brain meat contains omega 3 fatty acids, nutrients, and best for the nervous system. It is an antioxidant and helps to protect the human brain and spinal cord from damage.

Heart: The heart is a great source of Vitamin B2, B6, B12, and rich in folate, zinc, iron, and selenium, good to protect heart diseases as export says.

Risk of organ meat: Medical resources say that organ meats are high in cholesterol and saturated fats but new thought is that these two are important for a balanced diet but essential consumed in moderation.

There different methods to Improve food nutritious: Cooking method, Condiment, Groundnuts, Fermenting, Parching, Liming, Salad, Soup, Measurement

Cooking method;

Cooking effect on the chemical composition and its test, cooking makes food soft improve taste, kills harmful bacteria and parasites in meat and other foods. Proteins coagulated by heat. Vitamins are lost if too long to cook. Vegetables should not cook overheated and long. Eating raw and light cooking vegetables is an advantage. Cook on low frame heat. Cooking meat sterilizes the meat and kills parasites, meat should be cook on low heat, meat soup prepare on low flame it will take time to cook well and it good for digestion

Cooking is important for easy digestion; the human digestion system is not as strong as animals, for example, meat, animals consume their food raw, by cooking break its complex molecular structure into a simpler form. Some foods can chew and digest easily in raw form but some have to cook before eating. Do not fry; it involves a large amount of fat. Do not reheat repeatedly. Prefer to steam instead of boil. Fat-soluble vitamin D, E, and K are unaffected by cooking. Bacteria can killed by cooking.

Each culture and religion has its methods of cooking and is good. Cooking improves the appearance of several foods and makes foods more appetizing and palatable. Two methods can used in cooking; one is wet and the other is dry; in wet method cook under steam and boil and in second method food usually fry, roast, and bake, in the second method cannot lose lost of nutrients.

Condiments

Condiments improve flavor, color, and taste in meal. besides improving flavor stimulating the flow of digestive juices, condiments relieve flatulent distension that occurs from the fermentation in the intestine and well good for health such as black pepper, clove, cumin, chilies, turmeric, paprika, and coriander but these should be used as moderation if taken in excess tend to irritate and inflame the mucosa of the stomach.

Vinegar is also a well-known antiseptic and preservative. It softens the hard muscle fibers of the meat and the cellulose of green vegetables. It is also used for pickling fruits, vegetables, fishes and for preserving a small amount of onion.

Salad

For better health to start a meal with raw fresh salad includes fresh salad leaves, onion, cucumber, turnip, radish, carrot, cabbage, green coriander leaves, tomatoes, broccoli, and also can add some boiled bean but without bean can eat too. All vegetables contain minerals and vitamins. Beans are rich in proteins and Vitamins.

A fresh raw salad dish best to start a meal, Onion, tomatoes, cucumber, turnip, salad leaves, green chilies, broccoli, cabbage, carrots or other desire vegetables can add in a salad dish, veggies contain mineral and vitamins and best for health due to good nutritive value.

Groundnut; adding different nuts in different foods to improve flavor, nutrients and make a more delicious such as prune, dried apricot, almond, cashew, peanut, walnut, and dried grape may be eaten raw or used in cooking, brewing, and baking.

Note: Wash all vegetables thoroughly before cutting.

Fermenting

Making of curd of milk is one of the examples is fermentation. Some other food in which rice has fermented

Parching In this process, a puffing method applied to cereals like maize, rice, and wheat. Wet material is suddenly heated; the water escapes by puffing out the grain. Popcorn and murmur are parched products. Starch becomes more digestible in this process, cell walls of the starch grain ruptured and the large chemical, structures of the starch break down into smaller ones. Some loss of lysine in the protein does occur due to high temperature.

Liming

In most of the salad, items can add lemon or lime juice to in hence its taste and get Vitamin C too.

Soup

Soups provide nourishment as well as appetite and provide minerals, those prepared with meat stock rich in extractive, flavored. Soup can be prepared with veggies too.

Besides the above methods, most people use their cooking and presentation methods to make dishes more tasty and delicious, and delightful

Measurement

Keep a measurement utensil in the kitchen and add an exact amount of spices in the meal to it more delicious tasty and required quantity is also essential for health point of view.

 Here are measure charts so anybody can follow them to make food tastier.

Spoons

1 teaspoon is equal to 5 ml

1 tablespoon is equal to 15 ml

1 dessertspoon equals 15ml

If anything in 1 gallon that will be equals to 4 quarts, 8 pints, 16 cups, 128 oz, and 3.7 liters.

Other measurements are as follows:

1quart equals 2 pints, 2 cups, 32 oz.

1 pint equals 2 cups, 16 oz, 480 ml.

1 cup equals 8 oz, 240 ml, and ¼ cup equal 4 Tablespoons, 12 tsp, 2oz, and 60 ml.

1 Tablespoon equals 3 tsp, ½ oz, and 15ml. (tsp represents teaspoon)

Some other measurements are;

½ tablespoon equals ¼ tsp. 1 Tablespoon equals ½ tsp and ¾ cup equals 6 tablespoons, 2/3 cup equals 1/3 cup, ½ cup equals.

If anything is equaled to 2/3 cup it's half 1/3 cup is equal to 2 teaspoon and 2 tablespoons ½ cup half is ¼ cup and ¼ cup half is 2 tablespoon.

CHAPTER 4

Health

Most of the students/people ask me, what is health? What is the actual meaning of health? And what is a healthy lifestyle? Answers are not very simple because many factors are involved in one's health and lifestyle for example if someone is looking healthy by face, by work or by mental sometimes does not mean good health and sometimes does but in simple words, health is free from illness and injury or a person mentally and physically fit. The bad mental and physical condition indicates the unhealthy person or in other words, a healthy person means can perform his/her duties at home or other places well.

These facts that somewhere, some people, and sometime are not free from worries.

They are facing problem on every single day and also some persons are physically fit, emotionally no problems, social no problem, still environment health is there, I mean to say that there are somewhere some people are perfect and at the same time, somewhere some people are not perfect due to some reason.

This is also fact that everyone's health is in their hands, not always but sometime.

Everyone can be healthy if manage daily routine and make a plan.

 the plan means not necessary to write on a paper due to lack of time can ask someone to do so but this is important to maintain a task to achieve a goal if everyone does so then health automatically will remain good.

Health is all about good nutrition; good nutrition is essential for survival, mental development, physical growth, performance, and productivity. Some people say that health does not mean that someone looking nice, slim, doing work well fits from every angle, still, environmental problems and the surrounding atmosphere are there, the people are working in department have to manage it.

Health problem can solve using different techniques.

A person can improve by eating healthy, doing exercise, checkups to the doctor and keep away from stress, but still how to change the surrounding environment means pollution is there that is affected on the body, social behavior also affect on one's health and what you believe in, to solve all these problems is dependent upon everyone's responsibility. Every person doing a job, a job at home, out of home, walking, sitting, traveling everywhere a job, a job does not mean in a particular department so long in short, only a word responsibility is the solution of good health.

Home is that place where a kid learns a lot, from childhood for example' stay healthy means good nutrition if a childhood eats a full nutrient food from toddy that will influence whole life.

in short from a teenager, eating well will stay in good health later in life besides some worries and environmental health. A well-balanced diet is essential to insert into a habit. If a toddy does not know the taste of salt how he/she will add salt in their meal later so beginning should be for everything.

There are types of health as we all mostly heard and learn about x types of health, we will discuss ***Physical, Emotion, Mental, Environmental, Social, and Spiritual health.***

Physical health;

A person physically fit their body performance at work best, a fit person has sharper memory and less likely has depression, free of any injury can suffer hardship and ability to endure and good in breathing and heart function, muscular strength, flexibility, and body composition and well-being also help to reduce the risk of injury or any health issue. The body movement should be in the correct position of any sort of exercise. **Time of exercise;** morning is best for physical health. (If can manage 10 to 15 minutes) is a perfect time for physical health but if don't have time for morning walking can be managed in the evening before sunset or at night before going to bed. Physical health also depends on lifestyle, eating habits, income, and living environment, balanced diet, exercise, hygiene, and good sleep, to avoid unhealthy habits such as drugs, smoking.

Emotional health

Emotional health is an important part of our life. it is depend on family, friends and surrounding areas, living status, feelings, thought, and behavior.

When unfortunate things appear in one's life he/she becomes under stress obviously, stress effect on body weight, by increasing the levels of stress hormones (cortisol, intake) circulating in our body and these hormones cause us to have higher intensity craving for high fat, caloric foods, gain weight, skin bruises, muscle weakness, many health problems. Stressless eating food to make feel better such as dark chocolate, bananas and pears, black or green tea, yogurt, and food are containing soluble fiber.

If anyone controls emotion, thought, bad feelings, later in life it does not sign of a happy and healthy life could be a setback, but if eating stress less food can control easily. Improve emotional health in many ways, first to notice, what things are made angry or frustrate and sad, try to change those things but thing over and over before taking any step, if a matter is bothering first avoid if something happened and bothering you, keep busy yourself, change your surround environment if possible. Emotional eating is harmful because it causes weight gain at this stage your body does not need food. Studies have shown that a small amount of caffeine can boost brain function also stimulate the central nervous system.

Mental Health;

Mental health means that people emotionally, socially, and psychologically fit and perform daily activity in the best way. It affects, how we think, act, feel, and how to handle any situation, good or bad, stress, or stress-free. Mental health is very important at any stage of life. Good mental health means, dealing with everyone respectfully and kindly, take care of the ability to do anything in a good way. Keep a balance between work and play, activity, and rest. To keep the best mental health change situation causing stress at work and inactive condition.

Social health

Social health means the relationship of a person to other people, their families, friends, gathering, spending good time with other people.

A person's ability interact, appropriate relationships with other behavior, if a person socially active and has positive manners with others then will spend a happy life, necessary to learn how to deal with others includes our surroundings, family, and friend's behavior, in other words, social wellness is also being comfortable and to be able to engage with surround people. Social health is linked with physical health, socially healthy individuals are also mentally and emotionally fit, health will never face heart diseases, blood pressure, or any other health issue.

Environmental health

This type of health links to surrounding areas or atmosphere where we live, work, and daily activities performed it also includes air, water, source of food (should be safe), safe transportation, no pollution. To keep relax in any condition, enjoy with that thing, gives pleasure, do whatever want to do means no restriction at home, outside homework and other activity like playing a good game, watching favorites movie, listening music, reading a book, sharing feelings with a close person.

Spiritual health

Whatever people believe focus on it. it also teaches us the purpose of life, give some time for self-reflection, a spiritual person qualities are always thought positive, unconditional love, harmony, responsibility, justice, simplicity enjoy every movement of life. Do not interrupt others' believes. Spend some time with a positive person.

When anyone feels at peace with life then achieve spiritual health and it is that anyone can find hope and comfort in even the hardest time of life and spiritual wellness provides the system of faith, values, morals, beliefs, and principles and the practice of it may include fellowship, contribution, expression of compassion, belonging to a group, social contribution, volunteerism when we are spiritually healthy, we feel more connected to a not only higher power but those around us.

Spend some time in nature, practice gratitude, meditation, practice deep breathing, listen to different types of spiritual music Experts said that there is a close relationship between diet and memory. Get it easily on daily basis. Think about self-care; learn those benefits, which start from the beginning of the day. Eating healthy always to give favor to heart and brain keeping the body in good working order, essential nutrients for keeping the body healthy and in good working condition, eat more fruits and vegetable in balance. A good book is your best friend, reading a lot, keep busy avoid any negative thinking also keep away from stress. Salmon may be beneficial for reducing depression. Turmeric, dark chocolate, yogurt, green tea, citrus fruits reduce stress level, vitamin C is a powerful antioxidant that boosts the immune system as scientific studies show. If people will eat vegetables, all fruits, legumes, protein whole grains can reduce anxiety and stress. Banana is a good source of tryptophan, magnesium, and potassium in sweet potatoes help to reduce blood pressure and feel relax at the time of stress.

A balanced diet is essential. a healthy diet including all essential nutrients such as c proteins and high levels of vitamins, drink plenty of water, reduce stress, regular exercise, To use some other tips to help you calm down like breathe, listen to music, change your focus, start writing, drink green tea.

Green tea rich in polyphenols reducing inflammation and helping to fight cancer, help prevent cell damage and provide other benefits, reduce the formation of free radicals in the body, these radicals play a role in aging and all sort of diseases. The most important factor is to forget worries, stay cool, deep breathing, meditate on beliefs and exercise, to feel self-better write down feelings. Poor diet plays an important role to increase anxiety symptoms, headaches, digestive problems, and feelings of panic. Make a balanced diet chart; include vegetables, fruits, dairy, proteins, and grains in daily meals and snacks. Make time for things make to joy and make life healthy and happy also care for each other.

Keep brain young and sharp for life to avoid these foods include high fructose corn syrup and saturated fats, excess salty foods, sugary drinks. Study shows that high sugar diets can lead to a significant decline in cognitive function, altering long and short-term memory. Research also found that 6 to 9 alcoholic drinks a week can damage the brain. What we eat directly affects the structure and function of the brain and ultimately on mood.

The worst thing for health is fried foods such as French fries, according to the food export; artery-clogging fried foods increase the risk of Alzheimer's disease. Eating fatty fish per or twice a week, high fats cause fatigue. Garlic, reducing cholesterol, blood pressure, and antioxidant properties may reduce the risk of brain diseases. To improve mood and reduce anxiety, and depression, eat Selenium and fatty fish like salmon, sardines, mackerel, trout are high in omega 3, pumpkin seeds, dark chocolates, olive oil, turmeric, yogurt, legumes, chickpeas, beans, whole grains, avocados, and low-fat dairy foods. A good attitude toward other persons is essential for mentally disturbed people for mental health. A healthy lifestyle is not just eating healthy and doing exercise but to live with great respect. A healthy lifestyle is to spend a whole day without stress, worries, family, and circle friend's attitude. Emotional stress plays a very important in many illnesses, direct and indirect, most of the people feeling stress do smoke, over diet, overwork, sleepless, argue with others.

CHAPTER 5

Harmful effects on health

How to keep way from Germs, Drinks, Dietary disorder, Micro-organism, Food poison

Germs

Wash hand properly with soap. To remain neat and clean is an essential factor in human life to remain healthy. So wash hand before touching any food, any kitchen utensil should be neat and clean. Wash hand before start cooking and eating and after that. All cooking alliance should be washed before using, cooking and eating should be best, teeth should be clean before eating, mouth cavity perfectly alright. Germs remain everywhere so **health hidden in cleanliness**. Fruits skin should be neat and clean, bright in color.

Fresh and clean leafy vegetables;

Those are tender, bright green colored crisp free from insects, holes, and no mud in the leaves. Vegetable with a head like cabbage the hard heavy and compact free from worm and bruises are good and stored in cool and dry places and put in polythene bag when refrigerate. Wash all vegetables and other edible items.

Before cooking, grinding, chopping, cutting, or storing. Thorough washing is required to remove poisonous insecticide, spray, and egg of intestinal worms. Green leaves not cut into fine smaller pieces, this way loss of nutrients. Do not soak cut leaves for a long time, by doing so water-soluble Vitamin B and C will dissolve in water and wasted.

Boil water first then add vegetables instead to cook in cold water and then bringing to boil. If adding any acidic substances such as lemon or tamarind juice or sour buttermilk whenever will reduce the destruction of several nutrients like Vitamin C. Don't cook in excess water and avoid overcooking, reheating to avoid Vitamin C loss. Steaming vegetables is better than boiling.

Drinks

The best drink is mineral water while soft Drinks contain carbon dioxide, citric acid, and sugars. Fruit juices are noncarbonated drinks, citric juices contain Vitamin C while mango with milk is nutritionally very rich, and mixed fruit juices are healthy juices. Non-fermented drinks commonly used are Tea, Green tea, Coffee, Syrup, and Cocoa.

Fermented hard drinks are Alcohol, Wines, Beer, and Whisky and derived from a plant such as barley, rice, maize and grapes.

The food value of alcohol within limits; is a non-nitrogenous food and is a ready source of energy it is quickly absorbed from the gastrointestinal tract, requires no digestive process and utilized rapidly does not serve as reserve food, generally gives 7 calories but no Vitamins or minerals. When taken with other foods. The slow speed of drinking alcohol does not produce high blood concentration because as the alcohol is being absorbed time permits it's being converted into its break down products in the liver and rapid drinking of alcohol leads to high blood levels. Alcoholic drinks taken on an empty stomach is absorbed rapidly when taking food with drinks delays absorption and blood alcohol level remain lower by 30 to 50 percent. When alcohol taken before food works as an appetizer.

Effect of alcohol on different body systems

Central Nervous System, circulation, respiration, gastrointestinal tract, and kidney have effected by larger doses of alcohol. Exports say the manifestations of alcoholism depend upon the dose.

The nature of the environment, and on the inherent mentality of the individual, and would produce quite diverse symptoms on different persons and different effects on the same individual under different conditions. In moderate doses, alcohol acts as an analgesic by raising the pain threshold and induces sleep due to its hypnotic action.

When drinking a small dose of alcohol about 1 ounce produces a feeling of mental and physical well-being. Imagination becomes brighter and feelings are elevated, this first stage of intoxication, but the critical faculty dulled. If the dose is increased the intoxication observed where one loses self-control, but a confirmed drinker may hide it. The person will be talkative, sentimental, boisterous, or melancholic according to his peculiarities. Aggressive sexual behavior, emotion, imagination, and power of speech are excited. If the indulgence is continued further symptoms of acute alcohol poisoning appear so that the mental balance is lost. Talk, laughs, sings, and cries without restrain, but afterward loses control over these functions too. Speech becomes incoherent and at last, it is suspended after these muscles get affected, writing is abolished and if the dose is very large there is completely insensible, narcosis, muscular relaxation with the involuntary passage of urine and stool. Respiration is a slow, noisy, and shallow increase in pulse rate; it produces an increase in cardiac output for a short period and blood pressure slightly raised to maintain the circulation after peripheral vasodilatation. It produces a feeling of warmth, mild perspiration, and flushed skin especially of the face and temperature may low due to the effect of breathing and cyanosis and finally, the patient may die.

Dietary disorder
When people unable to get enough food, they remain undernourished, weak, and lack resistance against diseases.

We must take essential nutrients diet, improper nutrition leads to malnutrition, if a person eating carbohydrates, which provide sufficient energy in form of calories but in the absence of other essential nutrients certain metabolic abnormalities may also cause malnutrition. Malnutrition is a serious condition that happens when the diet does not contain the right amount of nutrients. Improper or inadequate food intake or may result from inadequate absorption of food. Natural foods are better for health. Oil should not exceed. Avoid eating deep-fried foods. Too many spices are also harmful if intakes daily. Do not eat salty foods. Several skin problems like acne, blackheads, pimples, premature aging, etc occur due to dietary disorders.

Micro-organism

Our earth is populated with countless organisms, these tiny organisms are so small that they can only be observed under a microscope, they range from simple microscopic to organism which is very large and complex, great variation in their form, type of nutrition, reproduction and the place in which they live. These tiny organisms are so small that they can only observed by microscope. They are usually simple in their structure and way of life. Microorganisms are viruses, bacteria, few algae, and all protozoa and many fungi, all are too small seen by the naked eye.

These organisms affect the welfare of humans, some of them are useful most of them are harmful.

Viruses

The word virus means poison. They are too small and cannot seen by a light microscope. They can study only under the electron microscope or through a biochemical test. All viruses are 10 to 100 times smaller than bacteria. Bacteria measure 1 micron = 0.001mm in size and are of many different types and shapes; round, rod-like, and crystal-like. The body of the virus consists of a central core of deoxyribonucleic acid DNA. In a structural view, they can consider neither animal nor plant. They increase in number by reproducing themselves like all living organisms. The properties and the presence of DNA is a positive sign in a virus. They can crystallize as a property of nonliving material and in this form, they can be stored for an indefinite period, without any loss of reproductive ability, and in favorable condition, they again start reproducing. Due to the properties of living and nonliving things, the viruse considered as an evolutionary point of view on the border of living and nonliving things. Viruses depend on other organisms for their nutrition and are invariably parasites on them. No organism is safe as they cause diseases in all organisms from bacteria to large animals, such as inhuman, they cause cold, smallpox, measles, polio and other diseases. In-plant they cause damages to leaves like in tomatoes, cauliflower, and potatoes, tobacco and others.

Bacteria

These are unicellular organism about a macron in size, most of them have no chlorophyll in their cells and heterotrophic can make their food and some are autotrophic bacteria cannot make their foods. Some of them are parasitic bacteria and live inside the cell of the animals and plants where they produce toxic substance and they are responsible for many animals and plants diseases, in human common diseases are **pneumonia, tuberculosis, diphtheria, cholera, and tetanus**, some bacteria are useful to make milk to yogurt or curd, cheese and sugarcane into vinegar.

Fungi

Fungi planted which lack chlorophyll and cannot make their food. They obtained their nutrition either from other organisms that live as parasites or as saprophytes by decomposing dead organisms. Some of the fungi as yeast are unicellular and microscopic other fungi are large and visible with the naked eye. The common fungi types are Mushrooms, Puccini, Mucor, Puccinia, Penicillium, and Rhizopus. Some of them are useful such as Penicillium for medicine and some are take in food like a mushroom.

Algae

Algae are the simplest plant and occur in both fresh and seawater, some algae found. Ninety percent of photosynthesis occurs due to algae, they are as the food chain serving as the food for the animal.

Oxygen produces during photosynthesis used by animals and plants by respiration.

Food poisoning

Microorganisms occur everywhere in nature even in the food we eat. They are on the surface of our skin and everybody's parts. The microorganism is associated in a variety of ways, with the food we eat. They may spoil the quality, availability, and quantity of our foods. Food serves as a medium for their growth. This growth causes food to undergo decomposition and spoilage. Some diseases produce microorganism release some toxic products, which get into our food and cause food poising when we eat it. Food poisoning may occurred by food taken infected with certain harmful bacteria. Food poising is characterized by gastroenteritis of abrupt nature due to ingestion of food or drink, arising either from intoxication or infection with either living bacteria capable of setting up the acute inflammatory condition of the alimentary tract or toxic substances produced by certain bacteria which have an irritant effect on the gastrointestinal mucosa. Food may become harmful due to the presence of bacteria.

 Frozen foods once thawed should not be frozen again for future use bacterial growth is increased in that case and when we eat it again food poisoning occurs. It is, therefore, necessary to protect the food from microbial contamination and spoilage.

Killing of micro-organism

Microorganism can kill by high temperature and Radiation.

High temperature

High temperature is most effective in killing these microorganisms; it can use by dry heat to use the oven or moist heat, where it is combined with high moisture. Moist heat is more rapid and effective; it kills these organisms by destroying their proteins. There are well-known methods to kill microorganisms but from those boiling and steam under pressure methods of moist heat are more rapid and effective and kills these microorganisms by destroying their proteins and spores.

Boiling, Steam under pressure, Sterilization, Pasteurization

Boiling:

In Microorganism most of the pores killed by boiling moist heat within 5 to 10 minutes.

Steam under pressure:

This the form of heat used in a pressure cooker, in different steam pressure these organisms can be killed within 0 to 15 minutes, steam under pressure provide heat higher 100-degree centigrade, steam can be reached inside material and killed micro-organisms

Sterilization

In this method of killing organism milk and fruit juice and other food products heat at 150 degrees of centigrade for 1 to 2 seconds to kill all microorganisms and spores. This method does not require refrigeration can be stored at room temperature for many days or even months.

Pasteurization

French scientist Louis Pasteur was discovered this technique, to use this method microorganism killed to heat control. In this process, the heat is controlled which kills most organisms, an example is pasteurized milk, to heat milk at 62.8 degrees of centigrade for half an hour or 71.7 degrees centigrade for 15 seconds in specially designed equipment. This sort of milk kept in the refrigerator to check the growth of those organisms to survived pasteurization.

Prevention of contamination: Contamination by microbes can prevent by preparing food and handling it in hygienic free conditions.

Preventing microbial growth and Slowing down metabolism

Growth and metabolism can stop and retarded by various means.

Chemicals, Dehydration, Low temperature

Chemical

In this way, food cans preserve by the addition of different chemicals such as acetic acid, benzoic acid, and lactic acid (vinegar). Pickle preserved by these organic acids. The acid lowers the pH and bacteria cannot grow.

Fungi and yeast;

Fungi and yeast not affect and may grow.

Dehydration

Dehydrates the foods by the sun or by heat to remove water, due to lack of water microorganism cannot grow. This is not necessary to kill microorganism but food does not spoil. Many foods such as prawns, fishes, vegetables, fruits, and meats, and others preserve by applying this method. Some foods are dehydrated by the high concentration of salt and sugar such as jam, jellies and honey, salted meats, condensed milk, and salted pickles due to lack of water the micro-organism cannot grow again.

A low temperature; Temperature at 0 degrees centigrade or lower retards the growth and metabolism of those organisms, but they are not killed. Refrigerators and freezers have improved the quality of preserved foods.

Several diseases caused by **microorganisms**, some of them are important to know everyone.

Some of the diseases due to bacteria are as follows:

Typhoid, Tetanus, Tuberculosis, Cholera, Bacillary dysentery

Typhoid

This disease caused by a bacterium salmonella typhi affected person continuously suffering from fever, headache, and inflammation of the intestine. The germs of disease enter the intestine of the human body along with food water; if an affected person once develops natural immunity against it the second attack in the same person is very rare, typhoid vaccine also is used to develop immunity in an affected person.

Tetanus

Tetanus caused by a spore-forming bacterium called clostridium tetanus, this species found all over the world. It found in umbilical stumps of a newborn baby, surgical suture and other injuries, deep wounds by rusty metals, nails are particularly dangerous. If the condition is anaerobic then these spores of microorganism germinate to produce toxin. The toxin affects the central nervous system and produces painful and violent contraction of body muscles. When muscles of the jaw are affected then the mouth cannot opened. The person said to have a lockjaw. Death results from respiratory failure. Tetanus controlled by immunizing the affected person with a vaccine that stimulates the body to produce antitoxin. For treating the patients, tetanus antitoxin is given to neutralize the toxin. Penicillin is given to stop the growth of bacteria and the production of toxins.

Tuberculosis

This disease caused by the bacteria mycobacterium tuberculosis discovered by Robert Koch in 1882. The symptoms of this disease are chest pain, fatigue, prolonged coughing, constant slight fever, and loss of weight. The sources of this disease are cattle and humans. The major causes of disease, living in a poor hygienic condition, dust, poor food, laden air, bad housing, and overwork.

The germs of diseases transferred from diseased person to healthy one either through the air in droplets resulting from coughing or sneezing or in foods handed by a person suffering from tuberculosis. The use of antibiotics is effective in controlling the disease.

Rest, fresh air, well regulated balanced diet can restore health in case of mild infection. Tuberculosis can be controlled to an extent by improving the work and living conditions of the people. Isolation of tubercular patients in hospital and sanatorium can control the spread of diseases to other persons.

Cholera

Cholera is a very serious infectious disease of the digestive tract caused by the bacterium vibrio comma. Cholera generally erupts in epidemic during rainy seasons or after the floods in any region as the water and other foods, stuffs become contaminated. The bacterium can transmit by contact with water and contaminated with feces from affected persons. The incubation period of cholera varies from a few hours to about 3 days. Symptoms of this disease are vomiting and profuse diarrhea type motions cause severe dehydration, loss of minerals, and increase acidity in the blood of the patient. Severe attacks may even lead to death in 2 to 3 days. The disease can control by active immunization of the population by vaccination with the cholera vaccine.

Water and foodstuff consumed should be clean and hygienic. Feces of the patient should be properly disposed of the patient to prevent the spread of the disease by flies.

Bacillary dysentery

This is a disease of the intestinal tract, caused by the bacteria of Shigella. The bacteria enter the human body by contaminated food and water. The patients suffer from diarrhea. The stool contains blood, mucus, and pus, sometimes the patient gets a fever. Diagnose of this disease done isolating and identifying the bacteria from the stool of the patient. The bacteria spread by feces, food, dirty fingers, and flies.

Humans are the main source of infection; the disease control by personal hygiene, proper sewage, sanitation, disposal, and fly control.

Diseases by viruses

Some important diseases by a virus are Poliomyelitis, Athlete's foot, Measles, Ringworm

Poliomyelitis: It is also known as infantile paralysis. This disease caused by poliovirus. The virus enters the digestive tract through the mouth, from where it penetrates the blood vessels finally reaches the nervous system, where it destroys the nerve cells and causes paralysis. The initial symptoms are fever, headache, stiffness of the neck and back paralysis, indigestion and vomiting, and spasm of a muscle.

The patients suffering from poliomyelitis should be isolated and immediately hospitalized.

Physiotherapy treatment applied to restore the activity of affected muscles. Infection transmitted with nose and throat discharges and feces. Children can immunize against this disease with the polio vaccine.

Athletes

It is the infection of skin and nails caused by a fungus belonging to the dermatophyte group. The skin starts peeling and cracking, nails get infected becoming yellow, thick, and brittle. The disease spread by person-to-person contact or by infected objects like towels. Excessive heat and sweat inside the shoes favor the growth of fungi. Toes get infected and itching between toes starts. The physician consulted for help as soon as the infection first detected.

Measles

The disease occurs due to the virus, which enters the human body through the respiratory tract. It enters the bloodstream; the measles virus causes cough, headache, and inflammation of the eyes. Spots in the mouth are present for several days before the rash comes out and diagnostic of measles. The patient is often very ill. The rash of measles consists of pink brownish blotches spread all over the body. After few days this disease begins to fade but staining of the skin may vanish after a week or two. The temperature also falls after a few days and by the end of the week, the patient feels well again.

The disease affected adults more seriously than children. No specific treatment for measles disease but antibiotics often used to prevent secondary complications.

Ringworm

This is an infection caused by a group of fungi belonging to the genus trichophyton. The fungi cause this disease. Another name of this disease is dermatophyte. The fungi attacking the skin cause localized lesions in the skin. Lesions assume circulation form as the growth of the fungus in the skin is more or less in all directions. Some dermatophytic fungi infect the hair follicles, nails, and hair. The fungus lives in the epidermis causes infection in the drier part s of the skin. Treatment is to use fungicide ointments for external use.

Diseases cause by parasites

Some common and important diseases by parasites are malaria, enteroviruses, and ascariasis. Malaria caused by a protozoan called plasmodium, injected in the blood of the human by mosquitoes.

In a malarial attack, the patient's body temperature is very high he/she feels cold. Attached is accomplished by nausea and headache, a few hours later the victims feel better though weak and tired, f patient does not get any treatment, they attack after every two or three days for several weeks before they get rid of this disease but without medical care, the victims may become sick again.

Some other dangerous and wells known as common diseases have been spread by viruses every year all around the world

Microorganisms have some useful aspect for us

Microorganisms used for the production of yogurt, cheese, wine, pickle, and beer. Many antibiotics obtained from some microorganisms for treatments of diseases. Microorganisms have used to provide antibodies on a commercial scale, which used against specific diseases such as cancer. Penicillium, Streptomycin, and tetracycline produced by different species of streptomycin. They used in the production of a vaccine. Vaccines used to immunize against diseases like tuberculosis, cholera, typhoid, measles, and other diseases. Some of the microorganisms produce vitamin B12, which used for treating anemia and as a food supplement. They decompose dead organic matter and convert it into nutrients. They used in sewage treatment plants to decompose the sewage.

These organisms increase the fertility of the soil by converting atmospheric nitrogen into nitrogen compounds, which can used by the plant for their growth. Some bacteria made to produce such hormones as human insulin, treat diabetes.

Boost immune health:

To improve the immune system change dietary and living lifestyle may strengthen the body's natural defense and defenses and help you fight harmful pathogens first of all get enough sleep to increase immunity, study shows those who slept fewer than 6 hours every night catch colder as compare those who slept 6 or more than six hours per night, getting adequate rest may strengthen natural immunity. Adults should get 7 or more hours of sleep and teens need 10 hours and infants and younger children should sleep 14 hours. Limit to watch TV, mobile screen time one hour before if you have any sleeping trouble as exports say or sleep in a dark room and also sleep at the same time daily. Eat more whole plant foods, healthy fats like omega-3 fatty acid and olive oil, and these oil naturally combat illnesses. Fermented foods such as yogurt, eating more sugar increase obesity, stay hydrated. Avoid eating unhealthy food on daily basis such as red and processed meats, Trans- fat, sodium, and sugar-sweetened beverages. Unhealthy foods are pastries, white rice, white pasta, fruit juice, wafers and snakes, white bread, bad fats.

Now a day's unhealthy foods high glycemic load includes many refined carbohydrates, soft drinks, cakes, white bread biscuits and high cholesterol foods like white bread, French fries, potatoes chips, industrial oils, pastries, margarine, Junk foods, all sugary drinks, cakes, and cookies are very popular, these foods expensive too. When you eat unhealthy food you can face lots of physical and mental health issues and will spend lots of money on treatment, a diet with a Tobacco medical sources say the impact on heart disease, stroke, chronic respiration, risk of cancer, and cardiovascular disease will increased due to an unhealthy diet. Seafood, under pollution, chemical use wastewater and biotoxins to avoid all these if you want to live a healthy long life. Avoid junk and processed foods like pizza, fried potato chips, and foods high in saturated fats ice cream, cake, and pastries sugary drinks. Study shows that consuming high levels of trans-fats hydrogenated oil especially can diminish cognitive ability and may cause brain shrinkage later in life. Certain high carb foods such as white rice and other bleached grain products have proved that affect mental health.

Avoid to eat unhealthy food on daily basis, in other words, fast food, snack foods packed calories, unhealthy fats, sodium, little or no dietary fiber highly processed foods tend to be low in nutrients and high empty calories due to refined flours, sugar, and sodium. Cheesy fries and other food high in fats, salts, fizzy drinks, frozen meals, and chicken nuggets are unhealthy.

Exercise

Exercise to keep the body active. What is exercise? In very simple words, the movement of our body at a greater intensity than the usual level of daily activity or in other words, any bodily activity that enhances or maintains physical fitness and overall health and wellness. Exercise can manage at home too. Exports give different names of exercise like Endurance activities; it increases breathing and heart rate. This kind of activity can reduce the risk of cardiovascular disease, type 2 diabetes, and high blood pressure may be lower the risk of cancer. Running, Swimming and dancing is an example of it. Another exercise is called Strength; makes body muscles stronger. Examples are cycling, dancing, and climbing stairs, lifting weight, working with resistance bands, heavy gardening (digging and shoveling), Push-ups, sit-ups, and squats.

Exercise stretches muscles and can help the body stay limber; examples are hiking, dancing, walking upstairs, tai chi, yoga, lifting weights. Walking backward, Walking heel to toe in a straight line, standing on one leg at a time, both lower body and core muscle strength, and standing from a sitting position is called balance exercise. These types of activities keep the cardiovascular system active and reduce the risk of cardiovascular disease, diabetes type 2, and high blood pressure, and maybe even lower the risk of cancer.

Exercise time

Early in the morning, the best time for exercise, walk-in front of your home or in a nearby park or any open space, if you do on daily basis it becomes a habit but its depend on everyone's getting time to do so.

Children learn most health-related behavior from the adults around them and parents whose play role model, eating healthy, and exercise habit tend to pass these on.

Benefits of exercise: Exercise can help to burn off extra calories and make you feel good. Exercise can boost heart health and strength. Our daily activity also burns calories (I count all my daily activity in exercise) walk at 4.5 miles an hour burns 150 calories. Running at six miles an hour burns 300 calories. Computer work burns 41 calories. Sleeping burns 19 calories. Swimming burns 180 calories can eat grilled chicken with vegetables. (For evening exercise)

Eat oatmeal with banana and almond after morning exercise; eat Salmon with sweet potato and vegetables after morning and evening exercise. Egg omelet with sweet potato can add desired vegetables and beans. Healthy homemade eggs with beans and salad also provided energy after morning exercise.

Healthy children's lunch

Remember do not forget kid's health. If kids will remain healthy, city will be healthy and the country will remain healthy. Beautiful kids usually do not like vegetables. You can hide vegetables with another delicious edible item like almond milk with almond butter, bananas, raw cauliflower, and beet and make smoothies. I am writing here some other smoothies and weekly lunch ideas and I'll write complete recipes in my recipe book and show them in videos on the YouTube channel or maybe on the website.

Some other smoothies are 1 cup orange juice or any other citrus fruit juice mix with spinach juice, cacao, dates, and mint extract or 2 cups milk with rolled oats, avocado, chia seed, drop of any syrup. Or 2 cups watermelon, raspberries, kiwi, broccoli, cashew, and maple syrup. Or 2 cup yogurt with rolled oat, berries, almond butter, chia seeds, and kiwi.

Weekly lunch ideas for kits

Theses some ideas, everyone can make as own with fruits/vegetables

Weekly lunch box idea for busy mom:

First day Monday; Brown bread toast with egg fried and apple.

Second day Tuesday; Brown bread pizza and mango slices or another season fruit.

Third day Wednesday; One cake piece or boiled egg, home fried potatoes, and blue barriers or other barriers.

Fourth day Thursday; Chicken boiled piece with black pepper fruit.

Fifth day Friday; Mix fruits and one small beef roast.

Sixth day Saturday; Tortilla rolls chicken and vegetable pieces and fresh juice or bananas shake.

7th day Sunday; Salmon fish piece and light sauce or

Remain healthy during all seasons

Vegetables and fruits eat every day whatever is the season and stay healthy in all seasons. First of all water; water is the best to keep dehydrates during hot summer. Add some cold juices and eat watermelon, cucumber, salad, smoothies, and lemons, and when it's hot out to avoid dehydration, skin sensitivities, and Vitamin and mineral other deficiencies also eat fresh fruits.

In the summer, eat Zucchini, which heat healthy and lowering cholesterol due to containing fiber pectin, watermelon, and full of water and fluid needs when the heat is on. Dark green leafy cold juices are good in the summer season.

Vegetable juices in summer

Water is essential for the movement of nutrients and dehydration occur due to the lack of energy, iron deficiency may cause fatigue, low energy, and irritability. Spinach rich in iron other foods like dark green leafy, seafood, poultry, peas are also rich in iron and best to consume vitamin C, peppers, broccoli and meals are full of vitamin C and iron. Watermelon keeps cool and hydrates in summer and its containing lycopene too, which protects skin cells from sun damage as experts said. Watermelon juice, orange juice, green leafy juice and soup, and tomato juice, yogurt, blackberries and raspberries, apple, pear, or any other fruits juices can be prepared. Stay healthy in winter with cold and flu season, exercise increase blood circulation and blood flow throughout the body, support immune system, diet that are rich in vitamin C, iron, Omega 3 fatty acid, potassium, and calcium. Everyone should be included green vegetable in everyday meal either in raw or soup, they are rich in vitamin A and C, iron and calcium low in calories and eat their roughage, roughage help to the movement of the wastage through the intestine tract and best to obese person and they are alkaline. Green vegetables help to keep weight maintain.

Eat sweet potatoes, carrot with both soluble and insoluble fibers. It is excellent for weight loss, butternut, and beetroot, oranges, fishes, eggs, and foods with beta-carotene, our body can convert beta carotene into vitamin A, which essential for skin health, vision, bone, immune, metabolism system and also is keep the mucosal linings in nose and lungs robust, to defend against infection in winter.

The U.S researcher said that too much beta-carotene can block some effect of vitamin A. Garlic and onion contains potent oil that has an antimicrobial action so they may help to protect against bacterial and viral infection. Drink tea without milk, lemon, and honey tea is anti-bacterial, and breathing in cilia to move out germs more efficiently. The cold and flu season made discomfort for most people due to the sneezing, headaches, sniffling but drinking an adequate amount of hot water helps to wash viruses and germs out of the immune system and keeps the body hydrated. They also support good gut health as periodic by promoting the growth of healthy bacteria. Eating vitamin C fruits and vegetables, vitamin C more doses perfect for people exposed to brief periods of intense physical stress such as endurance athletes or those living in very cold environments. Eat plenty of fruits and vegetables every day It give us enough vitamin C to support the healthy function of the immune system.

Eat enough vitamin D is helpful in respiratory infections by boosting levels of antimicrobial peptides, a natural antibiotic for lungs, eat oily fish that contain vitamin D, get from sunlight on the skin. Experts advise on buying and preparing winter foods that are good for health.

Winter healthy delight: All citrus fruits such as oranges, lime. Lemon, grapefruits, and legumes are healthy and hearty ingredients for winter, and of course, rich in important nutrients like fibers and protein

Winter vegetables; such as red and black beans, kidney beans, lentils, pinto, garbanzo cabbage and kale, nuts, cranberries and winter squash, turkey. All green leafy. Exports also say that winter squashes are also full of nutritional value; a cup of baked acorn squash cubes is packed with vitamins and minerals, 115 calories, 9 grams of fiber, 30% of the daily value of vitamin B-1, 25% daily value of vitamin C, and 31% of the daily requirement of magnesium included in only 1 cup.

Keep things in a better way

It is very important to know how to keep fresh foods and fruits without a refrigerator. To remove extra salt from curry, if curry becomes salty by mistake, then how to set it, do not worry. Make a small ball of flour and add in curry, boil curry for 10 minutes then remove these balls, curry becomes set. Or Drop a piece of white paper, white paper with absorbed salt, after 10 minutes remove from it. To store pickle for a long period, add lemon juice or apple cider juice, and mix well to remain vegetables fresh.

Sprinkle a few drops of apple cider on vegetables. Or Wet vegetables with water then keep them on paper. Or Wet thin cloth with water, wrap all vegetables. To keep fruits fresh sprinkle lemon juice on them. To remove fish smell; Some people do not like the fish smell, sprinkle 2 tablespoon salt on 1 kg fish, mix well and wash with clean water.

Eating a nutritious diet that has fresh fruits, vegetables, nuts, whole grains, proteins, and dairy will help maintain a healthy body, and it will help to regulate weight, vital signs, cholesterol, and immune system.

Conclusion

In this book, I have written on nutrition and health in detail try to clear that good nutrient has an impact on good health It essential to living, long and healthy life to catch a healthy lifestyle. A healthy lifestyle including each and everything should be in its proper range starting from cleanness, everything should be neat and clean. Knowledge of nutrients and their influence on health is essential to know every human being, to maintain eating balance diet implement it on daily basis. Essential knowledge of nutrients proportion is also important. Serving per/unit carbohydrate, fats protein, and mineral for in pregnancy, after blood donation, in some diseases, excessive menstruation, and infant growth.

Good nutrients are indispensable for health at all ages of life and satisfactory growth of infancy, childhood, and adolescence. It is the duty of every parent to teach their children from their childhood what balance diet, what foods are good for their health, and what to avoid eating. Do not eat only for taste and pleasure, eat for a healthy living most of the countries' people like more calories, not proteins, avoid those habit does not good for the body, balance diet s equal to balance health, balance health means there is no health error without a small single health issue. Health issues start from home.

Start the morning with hand washing, it just looks like a small thing but this the first step towards a healthy life, lots of bacteria and virus lives here and if a person eats anything without washing hand it will move towards mouth then in our stomach second is food washing and 3rd pots and place and so on. Long in short make a rule of healthy living and strictly follow that rule.

Nobody can insist on others do it and do not do it until and unless everyone gets to know themselves and healthy way to strengthen the immune system. Vitamin C is an essential vitamin to fight against viruses and bacteria; lack of this makes a person more prone to getting sick. Boost the immune system with the best nutrients to keep away viruses, infected bacteria, and live a long healthy life with a loving family.

Start the day with healthy eating one or two items regularly if want to live a longer and fully enjoy life with perfect health, less eating in the afternoon but that less should be healthy full of a nutritional valve in, perform small exercise daily either few minutes walking or another exercise depends on how much time you have. For those who love coffee does not mean drink unlimited cups; it opens the door for several potential skin problems that can dehydrate skin, magnifying the appearance of fine lines. If too much caffeine is interrupting sleep, the effects will show up on the skin while coffee does contain antioxidants, but too much could be on risk it on other hard drinks and irregular diet on irregular time.

Good nutrition diet including yogurt, oats, tomatoes, black beans, radish, walnuts, carrots, cucumber, and blueberries, pomegranate, grapefruits, strawberries, blackberries, oranges, lentils, and limes. There is some healthiest drink like coffee, green tea, low calories beer, milk, water, fruit juices, best low calories energy drinks, best green juices, you can get all from Amazon. You can prepare some green vegetable juice at home too. Apple cider vinegar is also a good weight loss drink.

Eating time maintain on everyone's needs. Malnutrition in many countries is more due to the ignorance about eating habits and lack of good nutrition and its link to health. Even well-educated people ignore a healthy lifestyle and also to avoid export guidelines.
Researchers say that the Mediterranean diet on traditional foods is good for health can cause weight loss and prevent heart stroke and diabetic type-2 and premature death.
Exercise and nutrition both very important, but remember at
At the end of the day, nutrition is the more important factor.
I will welcome if readers have any questions, suggestions, and write few words.

Glossary

Atherosclerosis: Hardening and narrowing of the arteries

Balance diet: A balanced diet contains all essential nutrients (carbohydrates, fats, proteins, Vitamins, and minerals) in a proper proportion according to the daily requirements of the body.

Cholesterol: Cholesterol is a fatty wax-like substance that the body needs to function properly but too much of it, that is bad

Fats: Fat is a type of nutrients

Fatty acids: Molecules that are long chains of lipid carboxylic acid found in fats and oil come from animal and vegetable fat and oil. Building blocks of fat in our bodies and comes from the food we eat.

HDL: High density of lipoprotein (good cholesterol)

LDL: Low density of lipoprotein (bad cholesterol)

Mole: Mole is the International System Base Unit of Measurement of a substance

Malfunction: Body function will not perform or purely body functions.

Protein: Protein is vital to life, it is required and repair cells and turn food into energy.

Retinol: Retinol is an essential component of the pigment Rhodopsin on which vision in dim light depends, to protector back of the eye layer (the retina)

Vitamins: Vitamins have named by using letters of the alphabet, the reason is when first discovered their chemical nature unknown

Vitamin B complex: (B1; Thiamin, Niacin, Riboflavin), (B6; Pyridoxine, Biotin), (B12, Folate)

Xerophthalmia: (from Ancient Greek) means dry eye, cornea produce, Xerophthalmia is a disease that refers to a constellation of ocular signs and symptoms associates with Vitamin A deficiency.

9 798502 398404